# Off
# Balance
## The American
## Way of Health

Dr. Leyla Ali, PharmD

Title: Off Balance, The American Way of Health
Subtitle: A Pharmacist's Perspective on why Drugs Don't Work
Author: Dr. Leyla Ali

Copyright © 2012 by Dr. Leyla Ali
First Edition, 2012
Printed in the United States of America

Cover Designed by Steven Peterson
Interior Book Designed by Kirsten Pederson

Library of Congress

ISBN   978-0-9853452-0-4

10  9  8  7  6  5  4  3  2  1

*The emperor walked beneath the beautiful canopy in the procession, and all the people in the street and in their windows said, "Goodness, the emperor's new clothes are incomparable! What a beautiful train on his jacket. What a perfect fit!" No one wanted it to be noticed that he could see nothing, for then it would be said that he was unfit for his position or that he was stupid. None of the emperor's clothes had ever before received such praise.*

*"But he doesn't have anything on!" said a small child.*

Hans Christian Anderson, *The Emperor's New Clothes, 1837*

# Dedication

To the ones I can count on to be there for love and encouragement
during the good, bad and ugly times: my sister, Dina; BFF Kelly
Dulin; Mother Diana (Gaga); and my dog, Jimmy.

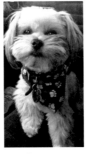

JIMMY

# Acknowledgments

This book started four years ago as a thought. After a journey of learning and crossing paths with the right people at the right times, the result is the creation of this book.

Several people were important parts of my journey. My deepest gratitude to:

**Chantel Zimmerman**, who taught the memorable classes "The Artist's Way" and "Vein of Gold," where I learned to let the writing flow through me.

**Sharyn Norwood**, my astrologer, who encouraged me to write this book back when it was barely a thought.

**Ted Strain**, for handing me my first cleanse and the book that changed my life.

**Richard and Sandy Stultz,** for welcoming Jimmy and I into your home for that week-long visit four years ago. This is where my writing journey started.

Editors **John Peragine, James O'Connor, Alanna Vitucci, Benedict Burns, Barbara Gibbons, Sharon Creal, Dina Ali Johns,** and **Kelly Dulin** came at the right time and added his or her own unique flavors and gifts to the book.

**Catherine Hawes**, my awesome researcher, editor, and all-around assistant extraordinaire, for all your hard work and dedication.

**Jeff Wheeler,** for creating my website, and providing continual support and encouragement.

**Steven Peterson,** for a sharp and brilliant cover design.

**Kirsten Pederson**, for hours of work and dedication which led to a bright and colorful layout for the book.

**Corne + Enroc Illustrations,** for taking my amateurish sketches and turning them into amazing cartoons that brought my ideas to life.

**Tom Gibbons, Nicole Baca, Dixie Stultz** and **Duncan Tooley** for their enthusiasm and support for this project.

**Dr. John Rush, Dr. Siva Mohan, Dr. Dennis Kinnane, Storm Cole, Art San, Raquel Reyna, Duncan Tooley, Sonya Aragon, Susan Moss, Frank Tortorici, Frank Ferrante, Bruce Miller, Dr. Robert Verkerk, and Peter Bedard,** my 14 interviewees, who all openly shared their journeys with me, and allowed me to share their journeys with the world. I love each and every story and I'm certain their stories will give others insight and inspiration as they did for me.

**Peter Bedard,** for creating the Alternative Healthcare Mixers and CreateYourHealth.com, where I learned so much and met many of the people who inspired or became part of this book.

**The Universe**, for lining things up so nicely and making me feel certain on my path even when things looked absurd.

# CONTENTS

# Introduction

Dr. Leyla Ali, PharmD

I didn't know there were choices. I didn't necessarily think that doctors and drugs were the best choice. I thought they were the only choice. I had never heard of alternative types of healthcare, at least not in a memorable way.

My father was a respected doctor and surgeon. Growing up, I experienced a prestigious and respected life thanks to his dedication to his patient's health. I grew up in a big house on a golf course with a view, which impressed our friends and visitors. At home, we had a cabinet full of medications and my siblings and I didn't have to wait long for a doctor's appointment. Our doctors were all friends of my father, and they helped each other's families with priority care.

My father ingrained in my two brothers, my sister and I that we would all go to college and become doctors. When I decided to go to pharmacy school, people told me it was a great idea and a good job, as I wanted to help people and work in healthcare.

From time to time I had heard that pharmacy "is all just a business," but I discounted those comments as made by bitter and negative people. In fact, I decided I would make it a point to never become like them! It wasn't until a few years after I graduated from pharmacy school that I fully understood what those people were talking about.

## APPROVED BY DOCTORS AND PHARMACISTS EVERYWHERE

Over the past 15 years, aggressive advertising by drug companies has manipulated the evolution of healthcare.[1] Today, doctors and drugs have become the standard, modern, superior, and even upscale response to any illness.

When I started school, my understanding of human health was pretty simple: if you're sick, the medicine cabinet had a solution. You needed to listen to your doctor and take the pills as prescribed, since doctors knew best. Furthermore, I trusted the doctors and the drugs, and I was relieved to know that I would always have access to both.

Today, it's not uncommon for patients to take a handful of medications on a regular basis.[2] One pill for diabetes, one for high blood pressure, another for cholesterol, a pill to heighten the mood when you're sad, and another to calm you down when you're anxious, an energy pill to get you through your day, and another to help you sleep at night, as well as others that your doctor has prescribed to treat whatever symptoms you are experiencing.[3]

It wasn't always this way.

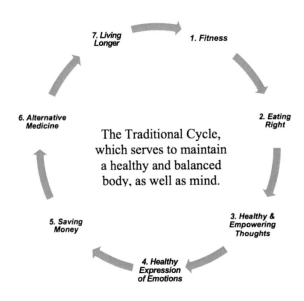

In the 1930s there were many more choices available. Patients could see any type of practitioner, including medical doctors, herbalists, homeopathic practitioners, acupuncturists, and others. These alternative medicine providers were considered an equal but different option to doctors and drugs.[4]

However, their status decreased and their presence faded inversely as pharmaceutical companies lobbied legislators to outlaw alternative medicine. This was done by creating regulations that made it difficult, if not impossible, for these holistic healthcare providers to stay in business.[5]

Additionally, the 1940s saw the development of penicillin and sulfa drugs. These *miracle drugs* treated infections completely and provided pharmaceuticals with a new platform to establish their trust and authority.[6]

In the 1980s the *wonder drug* Prozac was created[7] and in the 1990s, Viagra appeared on the market.[8] Each and every time a modern or miraculous drug was created, the public was mesmerized by the potential for a quick cure. This empowered pharmaceutical companies. The rush of customers made pharmaceutical companies rich, allowing them to advertise more, create even more drugs and pass more laws to protect their businesses.

This is the world that my generation was born into.

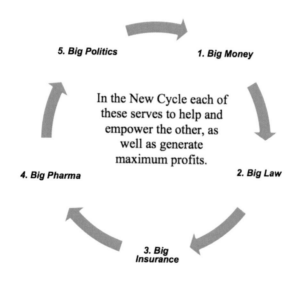

5. Big Politics     1. Big Money

In the New Cycle each of these serves to help and empower the other, as well as generate maximum profits.

4. Big Pharma     2. Big Law

3. Big Insurance

The new medical norm had developed into a delicate balancing act of:

1.  Providing cutting edge, new and exciting medications;
2.  Aggressively and emotionally marketing drugs through commercials; and
3.  Ensuring blind acceptance by the masses.[9]

I am not denying that doctors or drugs provide great benefit. It is important to give credit where credit is due. Doctors and the medicine they prescribe have made amazing progress in many areas of healthcare, from fighting infections to life-altering surgery. There have been drugs discovered that have kept people alive and surgeries that have separated twins conjoined at the head.

But I firmly believe that the medical profession has overstepped their boundaries. The medical doctors do not learn the limitations of their own practice, and will call certain health conditions "incurable" and keep the patient sick or on medications, when in fact alternative therapies can better treat the condition. Most medical doctors do not recognize or acknowledge the benefits of these alternative therapies, and the patients are the ones who needlessly suffer.[10]

The medical profession has degenerated from a healthcare system providing simple solutions into business system seeking profits. They now focus on treating the symptoms, not solving the medical problem. Treatments create long-term customers whose medical issues won't be resolved. And, the medications patients are prescribed? Eventually they too will lead to more medical issues, complications and side effects.

After all, if a drug company has experts test a drug, and the Federal Drug Administration (FDA) has approved the drug, and there are smiling and happy people on commercials that have taken the drug, then it surely must be good? I think many would be surprised at how those steps do not guarantee much.

When I learned these truths, I felt I had been betrayed and duped; as if I had dedicated my life to a scam.

My generation has never known a different world.

There is one more player in this game that I must identify—the insurance company. Insurance companies select which medications or treatments are covered for their members. They choose which product will be available to their members at an affordable price, and which pharmaceutical company will profit from their patients.

For some, it's easy to see that doctors and drugs are a system made for profits. For others like myself, it took a challenge and a journey before it became clear. Still, for most people, doctors and pharmacies are the only way.

They believe that it is the best, if not only, medical world that exists, so they accept the good and bad out of necessity.

Over the past several years, my perspective has shifted from a limited viewpoint as a pharmacist and doctor's daughter, to an awareness of alternative healthcare and its possibilities for health and healing.

I wrote this book to help you, the reader, understand that there are four pertinent realities when it comes to maintaining the health and vibrancy of your body, your mind and your spirit:

1. Although doctors and drugs are currently the accepted standard of healthcare in our society, they should only be one piece of the puzzle. They should represent one option, of many, working alongside other types of holistic healthcare providers.

2. Products that are displayed in advertisements are able to produce high profits, but are not necessarily the optimal choices for your health.

3. True health isn't a pill or cure waiting to be discovered. It entails going back to basics in terms of caring for your body, mind and spirit.

4. The realities and beliefs systems of our time have been molded by drug companies.

It's time for a paradigm shift.

In this book, I will share with you the history of doctors and drugs and how we came to this point today. I will also explore different types of conditions and show how western medicine's approach is vastly different from that of alternative medicines. Each chapter concludes with an interview, and many interviewees are ones who have struggled with their health and then sought, and benefited from, an alternative healthcare method. Some of my interviewees are holistic or medical practitioners.

There are many choices when it comes to our healthcare. Although many of us will rely on doctors and drugs for our healthcare needs, there are a variety of alternative and natural healthcare options available.

The idea of this book is not to push you away from doctors and drugs, but rather to provide a realistic viewpoint on the possibilities and limitations of doctors and drugs. I am not promoting one type of healthcare over another, but rather I want to present a variety of healthcare options and choices so that you can own your decisions, based on an understanding of what's best for you and your needs.

Dr. Leyla Ali, PharmD
2012

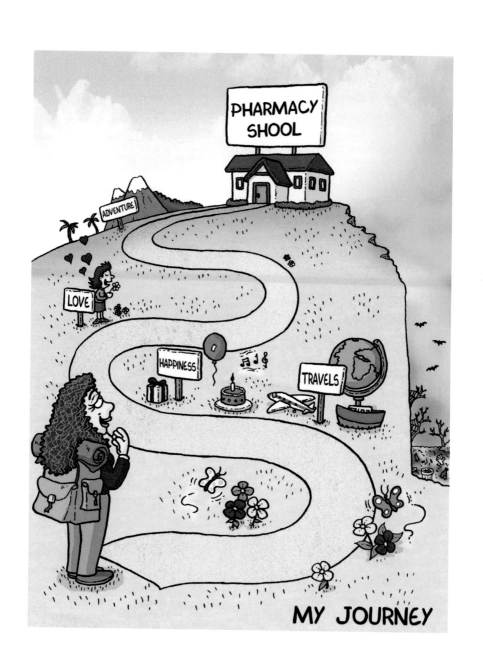

MY JOURNEY

## CHAPTER 1

# MY JOURNEY

*Every adversity, every failure, every heartache carries with it the seed*
*on an equal or greater benefit.* ~Napoleon Hill

Reflecting on my youth, I was motivated, energetic, optimistic—a dreamer. I imagined finishing school and doing something meaningful that would make a difference in the world. As frequently happens though, life had other plans for me.

My goal with this book is to share how I came to my point of view and shine the light on certain uncomfortable truths of American society. And, challenge you to test your own beliefs as it relates to the American medical system.

## MY JOURNEY

I was going to make a difference in the world by becoming a pharmacist. Instead, I have been schooled on the business of healthcare. And yes, make no mistake, it is a business. In fact, I have met others along the way who have come to same conclusion, but as a result of chronic health issues that are never cured. They only become long term customers of the healthcare system and pharmaceutical companies.

In 1991, I finished my BA in Anthropology at University of California, Irvine. While I certainly enjoyed the experience, after graduation I was a bit lost. I worked as a part-time delivery person for a local pharmacy, while I figured out what my next step should be. Oddly enough, a career in pharmacy didn't even register with me. Instead, I searched through graduate programs in Anthropology, thought about becoming a paralegal, and pondered the Peace Corps. But none of these felt quite right.

Then one morning, I awoke and I knew what I should do. I was going to become a pharmacist. It felt right. I signed up for two more years at the city college to round out my undergraduate education, and then applied to pharmacy school at the University of the Pacific in Stockton, California. In the end, I graduated as a *Doctor of Pharmacy*, and then started earning what seemed like huge amount of money, yet with over $90,000 in student loans.

Full of hope and excitement I started my first job as Dr. Ali, pharmacist. On day one, I was too slow on the store's computer system. On day two, I didn't answer the phone within three rings. During days three to five? I spent my time learning how to respond to endless questions that had nothing to do with prescriptions:

> *"Why doesn't my insurance pay for this?"*
> *"Why is my prescription taking so long to fill... don't you just pour some pills in a bottle?"*
> *"What's the holdup?"*

I had a Doctor of Pharmacy degree, $90,000 in student loans to pay back and I was essentially working a retail job. Instead of helping sick people get better I was completely bored and forced to endure a time clock. On day six I decided that I would be out of pharmacy work in three years, and it didn't matter what I did afterwards.

*Restless, depressed and exhausted* summed up this period of my life. It was my accountant, of all people, who helped me find meaning in my life again, when he off-handily recommended the book *Rich Dad, Poor Dad*[11] while reviewing my tax return.

I bought the book and was hooked. While reading it, I realized that I:

- Had fallen right into the trap of swapping days for dollars;
- Lost the hope to succeed financially or to gain true financial freedom;

- Gave away my time, and was living an unsatisfying life;
- Was using very little of my personal knowledge; and
- Felt like I wasn't really helping anyone anymore.

The book also sparked personal action— a lot of it.

Soon, I was involved in real estate, taking screenwriting classes, and learning about internet marketing. I was desperate to escape from retail pharmacy and find something personally and professionally motivating and rewarding. Unfortunately, I tended to shoot from the hip and jump into real estate deals before I was ready and with partners I hardly knew.

This sparked the next life lesson in my search for financial freedom and personal satisfaction, and it wasn't pretty. Five years after I started working in retail pharmacy I now had to deal with the following issues:

- Multiple creditors calling me at work, seeking payment on debts totaling deep into six figures;
- Two home foreclosures and a short sale;
- A real estate partner under investigation by the FBI; and
- A stress level directly impacting my job performance.

I took a hard look at myself and my situation and made two decisions. I resigned from the pharmacy with my secure comfortable salary, and filed for bankruptcy.

It wasn't until a few years later that everything clicked. I mentioned to a friend that I wanted to learn about cleansing and detoxification of the human body. My friend brought me a cleansing kit and explanatory book to read. I intended to only skim the contents quickly enough to get the main points. Instead I was captivated and read it cover to cover. *Cleanse and Purify Thyself* [12] by Richard Anderson, was one of the most enlightening and eye-opening books I had ever read.

It claimed that nearly 99 percent of known human disease is caused by what we eat. I thought to myself, *ridiculous! I am a Doctor of Pharmacy and of course I would know if this were true.* So, I dusted off my text books from pharmacy school, specifically, the primary therapeutics book used during my years of study, *Pharmacotherapy, A Pathophysiologic Approach.*[13]  I skimmed through, researching various diseases and the prerequisite list of causes.  A few items stood out:

- **Ulcerative Colitis.** "Although the exact etiology… is **unknown**… the major theories [include]… infectious or immunologic causes," (p. 733).

- **Acne.** "The causes of acne are multifactorial and are **not completely understood**," (p. 1816).

- **Gastroesophageal Reflux Disease.** "… is related to the **complex balance between defense mechanisms and aggressive factors**," (p. 31).

- **Asthma.** "Although a **single underlying cellular defect has not yet been discovered**… hyper-reactivity of the airways to physical, chemical, and pharmacologic stimuli is the hallmark of asthma," (p. 554).

- **Alzheimer's disease.** "Alzheimer's disease… is a type of progressive dementia for which **no cause is known** and no cure exists," (p. 1325).

- **Rheumatoid Arthritis.** "The factors that initiate the inflammatory process are **unknown**," (p. 1717).

For condition after condition, the causes in the text were listed as *unknown.* Yet the text presented calculations that identified populations where episodes of the disease may be prevalent.  In other words, Western Medicine, with all its research capabilities and technological advances, staked no claim in understanding causes.  Rather, the *solution* was in detailing treatments and prescribing pills in order to sway the statistics.  The answer lies, I realized, in treating the symptoms, not in discovering the cause of the illness and eliminating it.

All my years in pharmacy school had earned me the glamorous title of "doctor," yet had not taught about cleansing and toxins.

4

After discovering the shortcomings of current practices of Western medicine, I started to research alternative methods of treatments that yielded better results. It eventually became very clear to me that many standard medical treatments are manufactured in order to:

- Create long-term customers;
- Provide patients with temporary comfort; and
- Specifically, NOT treat the underlying cause.

This is because it is only when people become repeat customers that drug companies are able to create and enjoy great profits. In other words, *IF A DRUG COMPANY CAN AFFORD TO ADVERTISE THEIR PILLS OR PRODUCTS ON TELEVISION, THEN THEY ARE ABLE TO CREATE LONG-TERM CUSTOMERS, AND BIGGER PROFITS!*

Seven years beyond pharmacy school graduation, I've returned to the JOB (just over broke) scene. I was in bankruptcy from the results of bad partners and decisions in real estate. I still had $75,000 in student loans, and I was experiencing the ultimate insult—the awareness that I was trapped in a profession that I no longer believed in.

I had the wisdom and knowledge that I was not encouraged to share, and most pharmacy customers were not interested in anyways. Customers demanded their pills; they have no desire to hear about *alternatives* (which were seen as a bad word due to good advertising by drug companies). And, I was still filling prescriptions.

This brings me to the current moment in time with my desire to promote a better way of caring for one's health.

My training as a doctor of pharmacy did not teach me about the holistic view of human health. I did not learn in school about the direct connection between what we put in our bodies, both voluntarily and involuntarily, and the diseases which plague our society. The so-called experts are still trying to figure it out, yet in the meantime, powerful forces are defining all the rules.

To sum it up in one statement: *Relying on doctors and pharmacists for your complete healthcare is like relying on a pesticide expert to maintain your entire vegetable garden.*

My goal is to create a new awareness of the pitfalls in American healthcare, while also providing solid solutions to health conditions and diseases by offering informed choices. Empowerment and truth-filled knowledge is the first step.

But isn't Western medicine a good response to our fast-paced society? Americans are trained to seek a quick meal, a fast drink. Similarly, we need our medical solutions to be speedy, easy and miraculous. It's a sad reality, but many people do not search for alternatives until their medical condition becomes uncomfortable or hopeless.

More importantly, we need to recognize and change bad living habits into better ones. This is the best prevention to sickness, and an area I will focus on extensively in later chapters.

As I was moving along my journey of discovery, I met several people along the way who found their relief with holistic and alternative medicine. At the end of each chapter throughout the book I have included interviews with a variety of individuals, many of whom struggled with a condition or disease for years and found no relief with Western Medicine. When they discovered holistic health they were able to heal themselves. Several have changed the course of their lives to become holistic or alternative healthcare practitioners.

Many of us have grown up with strong faith in the medical system. It took me years to learn the disappointing truths that it doesn't have all, or even most of the answers. And, now I join the many who aim to help people find better ways to maintain and manage their health.

Western medicine will always be present and available for those who seek the next miracle drug. For others, I hope they will look at lifestyle adjustments and alternative forms of healthcare long before their health is compromised.

I hope my readers come away from this book with a deeper understanding that good health is a matter of mind (thoughts, beliefs and attitude), body (what goes in, how it's treated) and spirit (a desire to live happily, a connection to higher source), rather than the next pill.

And to remember, it's a process. It takes small steps to change habits, but doing so can fill your life with happy and healthy moments and years.

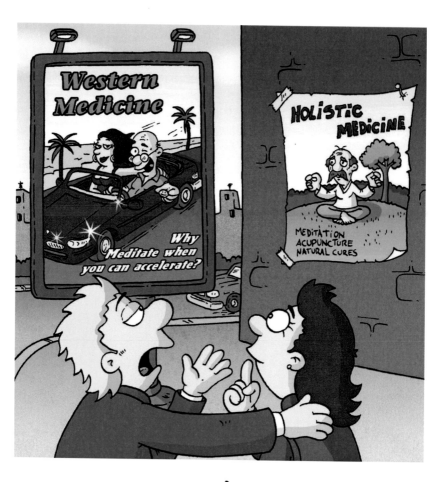

THEY CAN'T EVEN
AFFORD TO ADVERTISE !

## CHAPTER 2

# WHY WESTERN MEDICINE?

*There are always two choices; two paths to take. One is easy. And its only reward is that it's easy.*          *~author unknown*

My father was a doctor and my mother a surgical nurse. We always had access to healthcare and drugs, which included a medicine cabinet filled with prescription bottles. In fact, for much of my young life, I thought that this was the only type of healthcare. A college course, entitled Medical Anthropology, was the first exposure I had to alternative forms of healthcare.

Have you ever wondered about the origins of United States' system of medicine? After pharmacy school, I began to.

The *American Medical System* is considered the gold standard of healthcare; it is the envy of the world, and the standard response to illness or injury. American healing is based on the premise that "your doctor or pharmacist are the experts and will tell you" what to do.

But, we didn't begin with this mindset, rather our society has evolved to the point where there seems to be a pharmacy located on every street corner. In fact, today, our medical industry has become a *feeder system* for pharmaceutical distribution.

Many simply accept this as the best way, and therefore, it must be the only way. The truth, however, is that our options for health and wellness management abound in this country. However, the alternative and natural healthcare modalities sit in the shadows of powerful doctors and drugs.

## HOW DID THIS HAPPEN?

Why did our government choose this healthcare model? Was an exhaustive review and comparison of all the options completed? Why did naturopathic, homeopathic, and holistic procedures get shoved out of the way? When and why did they become *alternative*? Are pharmaceuticals, prescribed by doctors, the superior solution? Or, is this a direct result of our capitalist-based structure?

I wonder, is Western Medicine—with doctors and drugs—the norm because it is most effective? Or, is it because it offers an easy fix, and quick profits? If that is the case, is it any wonder healthcare legislation is heavily lobbied by the profitable and powerful pharmaceutical companies? Alternative treatments that cure, rather than treat illnesses, cannot compete and are minimized and trivialized.

## A BRIEF HISTORY OF MEDICINE

Since the earliest times, humans have relied on plants and what we now consider *alternative medicine* to treat illness and disease.[14] The Chinese developed acupuncture treatments 6,000 years ago in China, which offers cures for almost all medical problems.[15] Ayurvedic medicine, which matches treatments to an individual's body type and spiritual energy, began 5,000 years ago in India.[16]

More recently, the Egyptians, the Babylonians, the Greeks, and even the Romans, all treated their sick with herbal remedies. In fact, there were books produced in the fifth century BC[17] (at the time of Hippocrates, the father of Western Medicine) that illustrated flora and fauna as well as what illness each successfully treated. These books were later copied by monks in the Middle Ages, thus carrying the knowledge forward to the Renaissance and present day.[18]

During the Middle Ages, women were the keepers of this knowledge and healers in villages; although, many were accused of being witches and burned at the stake.[19]

The late 1800s saw an increase in migration from around the world to the US. These new citizens brought with them their traditional health practices that worked. In fact, until 1910, holistic therapies were taught in most medical schools in the United States, while only a few schools trained in the extensive use of drugs as therapy.[20]

## THE ERA OF THE AMERICAN MEDICAL ASSOCIATION

It is only since the early 20th century that we have depended upon doctors and drugs to address our illnesses.[20] The paradigm changed when John D. Rockefeller and the American Medical Association (AMA) hired Abraham Flexner, a high school teacher, to evaluate the effectiveness of therapies taught in medical schools around the country. In 1910 his findings were published in the *Flexner Report*, which denounced natural/holistic therapies and approved of and promoted drug-based medicine.[21]

The AMA was able to use the *Flexner Report* to argue before Congress that alternative medical treatments should be discarded in favor of western medical care. Over the course of the next 15 years, the number of natural and holistic schools plummeted from 600 to 50, while the number of AMA-approved programs increased.[20] Even more disturbing was the power given to the AMA to decide what is or isn't considered medicine. Since then, the AMA has worked actively to discredit and outlaw any form of medical competition: specifically holistic and natural therapies.[22]

The 1930s saw the discovery and mass marketing of penicillin and sulfa drugs[23], which in the 1940s, further cemented Western medicine as the most powerful way of treating disease. As more people became confident of Western medicine's potential, more businesses were created and more money was invested in research. The result of this was the consolidation of consumer healthcare and medical thought.

During this same period, two important treatments for cancer were suppressed by the Food and Drug Administration (FDA) and the AMA. The first was the *Rife Machine*. It was created in the 1930s by Royal Rife. Rife discovered that certain frequencies kill bacteria and viruses and was

**11**

using them to successfully treat his cancer patients. His machines were discredited.[24] In the 1980s several new Rife Machines were built and tested, and they achieved amazing results.[25]

Secondly, in the 1940s, Harry Hoxsey developed the *Hoxsey Treatment*. His cancer treatments consisted of a caustic herbal paste for external cancers or an herbal mixture for internal cancers, combined with laxatives, douches, vitamin supplements, and dietary changes.[26]

Within ten years, Hoxsey operated 17 alternative health clinics in 17 states. Thousands of his patients claimed that he had cured them of cancer. The AMA launched a vicious attack against him and he was arrested over 100 times. Every time he was thrown in jail, hundreds of his patients would surround the jail and sing and pray until he was released.[20] Over the next several years, the attacks on Hoxsey by the AMA and police departments continued. Finally, he sued the AMA for slander and libel, and he won. He was the first person to win a judgment against the AMA.[27]

After an in-depth investigation by the U.S. Senate Commerce Committee, it was concluded that the FDA, the AMA, and the National Cancer Institute *conspired* to suppress a fair investigation of Hoxsey's treatments. By 1953 his clinics were flourishing and he had successfully treated over 12,000 patients.

Unfortunately, in 1960, the FDA found a way to shut down all 17 clinics: they stated that there is no known cure for cancer and therefore that what he was doing was illegal.[20]

The 1950s, 1960s, and 1970s also saw a growth in chiropractic care and its popularity due to its widespread therapeutic success. This too disturbed the AMA, which in the early 1960 began an attack on chiropractors, as well as holistic and natural healers with the intent to shut down the profession entirely. Their public relations campaign included describing holistic, natural, and chiropractic care in magazines as a *fraud, hoax* or *cult*.[28]

A new interest in alternative healing wasn't born until the mid-to-late 1960s when the hippies and the yogis headed west, and the Beatles were publically exploring transcendental meditation and alternative medicine.

This created a tipping point, as more and more people began looking for an antidote to the Western medical tradition.[29]

From the 1970s to the present, more and more people have discovered alternative medicine; a greater percentage of the population of the US is either taking supplements or has partaken in some form of alternative medicine, including: acupuncture, chiropractic care, Chinese herbs, Ayurveda, yoga, homeopathy, and thousands more types of alternative healing.[30]

## MASS-MARKETING

The 1980s saw the development of a number of blockbuster drugs. First came Prozac, followed by Zantac, which was mass-marketed and became the world's biggest-selling drug in 1988. Then, in 1997 pharmaceutical ads were approved for television and radio.[31]

The past 15 years have been a constant barrage of television ads depicting picnics, big white fluffy clouds, and promises for magical medical solutions; all with exaggerated smiling faces that quickly mumble through an often long list of side effects. This change took the marketing of drugs to an entirely new level. Instead of doctors recommending medications, patients now requested and/or demanded specific medications from their doctor.[32] Additionally, In fact, between 1999 and 2000, the amount or prescriptions for the 50 most heavily advertised drugs rose six times faster than prescriptions for all other drugs.[33]

## AN UN-NATURAL EVOLUTION

In summary, Western medicine has evolved into the gold standard of medical care as a result of the creation of some profitable drugs and the suppression of alternatives methods.

While there have been some very good breakthroughs with antibiotics, other types of medications have created more sales and profits. Drug companies have used these profits to make themselves even more powerful. This, combined with the suppression of holistic and natural approaches by the

AMA (which works to promote the best interest and the profession of the medical doctor) has created a medical nightmare.

It has come to the point where the most *profitable* healthcare has become the standard and trusted healthcare. Meanwhile alternatives that offer cheaper, less painful, and more powerful treatment options have become disputed.

With the growing population and choices for healthcare, it's true that our government had to step in and organize, or provide, some regulations and standards for healthcare in order to keep out the fraudulent practitioners. However, the decisions made by the AMA and the FDA have generally been in the best interest of doctors, drugs and profits, not the health of Americans.

## SIDEBAR #1
## FDA Drug Approval

As a side note, for a drug to be approved by the FDA, the pharmaceutical companies must perform extensive, controlled studies. Typically, this involves randomized, double-blind tests; a group of individuals ingest the actual medicine while another set of testers take a placebo. None of the "guinea pigs" actually know whether the pill they swallow is real or fake (thus, random). Any of these new drugs are tested against placebos or other drugs.[34]

Yet there are no tests that compare the long-term use of drugs over alternative healthcare options. In addition, what are the different types of holistic health practices, and how do they work? Are there studies that compare how a certain health condition responds to drugs versus an alternative approach? There aren't many tests like these as there are no large corporations that serve to profit from these comparisons.

If you are like most people, these questions do not come to mind, and all the *research* is done for us. The American medical and pharmaceutical industry was chosen for us. In fact, many people spend more time shopping for shoes and flat-screen televisions than researching the different types of healthcare options available.

**14**

## Holistic Therapies versus American Standard Medicine

Doctors and drugs treat the symptoms and provide quick relief that fits in well with our fast-paced society. Why are there so many pharmacies? Probably for the same reasons that fast food chains are so successful. People are hungry and want a quick, cheap, and convenient solution. Pharmacies offer the same sort of benefits.

| The following are several key distinctions between holistic practices and the standard American (Western) medical regimen: | |
| --- | --- |
| **Holistic medicine...** | **American standard medicine...** |
| Treats the whole person, including integration, balance, and harmony of the physical, mental, emotional, spiritual, and social aspects of the individual. | Treats physicals and mental problems if they are disruptive to someone's life. |
| Treats the cause. | Treats the symptoms. |
| Seeks to do no harm. | Seeks to do no harm, in theory. |
| Believes the body has the power to treat itself. | Believes the illness is treated with a drug. |
| Views the physician not only as a teacher, but as someone who motivates and empowers a patients to heal themselves. | Views the physician as the writer of the prescriptions, and a good patient as compliant and willing to take the medicine as prescribed by his or her doctor. |
| Views prevention as the best method to health. | Believes in prevention, but doesn't really know how to prevent disease. |
| The primary goal of a holistic practitioner is to promote physical and emotional wellness. | The primary goal is to stabilize with medications and to profit. |
| Treats the entire person including body, mind and spirit. | Treats the part that is *broken*. |
| Focuses on what's right with you. | Focuses on what's wrong with you.[35] |

**What other types of healthcare exist?**

There are several other types of healthcare practiced all around the world, and some, like Ayurvedic medicine and Chinese medicine, have been in existence for over 5,000 years. The following is an abbreviated list of many legitimate forms of natural and alternative healthcare that exist:

---

### EXAMPLES OF DIFFERENT TYPES OF ALTERNATIVE AND NATURAL THERAPIES

**Acupuncture** is an ancient Oriental healing technique, especially utilized by the Chinese. It involves piercing pressure points of the body with needles to treat disease, relieve pain, and balance mental/emotional disorders.

**Aromatherapy** entails the use of therapeutic oils for stress reduction, deep relaxation and a variety of other means. Often used with energy work such as Reiki, massage, and meditation. An aromatherapy specialist makes up special mixtures of oil blends for a variety of healing purposes of the body, mind and spirit.

**Ayurveda** is the traditional Hindu system of medicine in India since the first century AD. The system utilizes a combination of herbs, purgatives, and oils to treat disease, and imbalances in the body and mind. The Ayurvedic system has categorized people into three basic body-personality types known as Vata, Pitta, and Kapha.

**Chinese Medicine** is unlike Western biomedicine that conceptualizes the human body as a bunch of assembled parts. The Chinese philosophy is more elaborate and sees the body, the world, and the universe as an interconnected whole. It is the diamond web where you pull one string and everything else is influenced.

**Color Therapy** is a technique that uses color and light to balance energy wherever a person's body be lacking, be it physical, emotional, spiritual, or mental.

---

**Flower Essences** are based in the Bach flower remedy system, and are used to treat a variety of emotional problems and challenges from anxiety, anger, depression, fear, hopelessness and entrapment to withdrawal, grief, abandonment, and loss. Tinctures are taken sublingually, or often as a soothing enhancement in a bath or massage.

**Homeopathy** is an alternative therapy in which practitioners use highly diluted preparations. Based the *law of similars*, preparations which cause certain symptoms in healthy individuals are given in diluted form to patients exhibiting similiar symptoms.

**Naturopathy** provides treatment and self-healing for a variety of diseases and ailments from the consumption of specified whole foods, herbs, spices, and plants.

**Polarity Therapy** utilizes positive and negative magnetics to balance chemical-emotions in the body. Treatment may include a variety of applications from foot magnets, healing rods, ionic hydrotherapy, and electrical stem.

**Qi Gong** is a Chinese form of healing that focuses upon moving energy through the body, combining exercises, breathwork, and meditations. Medical qi gong is a form of qi gong practiced only by a master and is used in healing applications with other forms of Chinese medicine.

**Reflexology** is a form of acupressure specifically focusing on massage and stimulation of such points on the hands and feet.

**Reiki** is an ancient form of energy healing. Modern Reiki practitioners have been attuned by a Reiki master to secret symbols that unlock the flow of the healing energy. They serve as the channelors of the energy to their clients. Reiki can be used for many purposes such as to shorten healing time, reduce or eliminate pain, and remove energy blockages that interfere with sleep, and therefore healing.

**Sound Therapy** is the use of sound and music for healing. Sound healing offers the possibility of a drug-free way of treating pain and illness.

**Theta Healing** is a holistic healing technique which focuses upon thought and prayer. Theta Healing relies upon The Creator of All That Is, allowing miraculous instant healings and profound transformations.

## POINTS TO REMEMBER:

- Doctors and drugs are the most well-known type of healthcare in our society because they advertise extensively on television, online, in newspapers and magazines, as well as on the radio.

- The fact that pharmaceutical companies are able to spend so much money to advertise merely demonstrates that it's a very successful business system with repeat customers; it doesn't necessarily mean that they are the best type of healthcare.

- Western medicine teaches the patient to listen to the authority of the doctor, whereas holistic or natural healthcare teaches and empowers patients to heal themselves.

## INTERVIEW WITH MEDICAL ANTHROPOLOGIST
## DR. JOHN RUSH

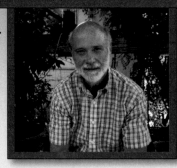

*John A. Rush, PhD., is Professor of Anthropology at Sierra College, Rocklin, California, teaching Physical Anthropology as well as Magic, Witchcraft, Myth, and Religion. He and his wife maintain a large herb garden where students and faculty learn about the cultivation and preparation of numerous medicinal and magical herbs in addition to the myths that surround them. Dr. Rush is also a retired clinical anthropologist and medical hypnotherapist in private practice from 1972 to 2008.*

*Dr. Rush's major publications include* Witchcraft and Sorcery: An Anthropological Perspective of the Occult *(1974)*[1]; The Way We Communicate *(1976)*[2]; Clinical Anthropology: An Application of Anthropological Concepts within Clinical Settings *(1996)*[3]; Stress and Emotional Health: Applications of Clinical Anthropology *(1999)*[4]; Failed God: Fractured Myth in a Fragile World *(2008)*[5]; and The Mushroom in Christian Art: The Identity of Jesus in the Development of Christianity *(2011)*[6].

**Dr. Leyla: What is a medical anthropologist?**
Dr. Rush: Medical anthropology is a part of the field of anthropology that focuses on how human cultures define and affect medical and health issues. As medical anthropologists, we often study topics such as healthcare culture and practices, cultural interpretations of medicine and disease, and cultural disparities in health and healthcare provision.

**Dr. Leyla: Please describe your activities as a practicing medical anthropologist.**
Dr. Rush: My practice involves holistic health, which means that I am interested in the cause of symptoms including emotional/relationship issues. As most health issues revolve around diet/nutrition and cellular toxicity

(not germs and bad genes), I take a complete health history and provide information on dietary problems and cellular detoxification. My specialties involve diet and nutrition, detoxification, cancer therapy, hormonal re-regulation, and aging. I also conduct individual, marriage, and family therapy as well as being a Certified Medical Hypnotherapist using hypnosis for emotional/physical issues. Finally, I use numerous symbolic techniques to signal cure and reintegrate an individual back to their group/culture.

**Dr. Leyla: What do you see as medical anthropology's major contribution to the understanding of the processes of health and disease?**
Dr. Rush: This would be the comparative process, which shows us that cultures, for the most part, engage in the same healing processes. The content, however, changes from culture to culture. This comparative process also shows that, in the West, we are not as interested in health as we are in illness maintenance (there is no money in health). We treat the individual as separate from the culture, and there is no signal to cure nor is there (usually) social reintegration of the individual back to his or her culture or group (this is especially the case in clinical psychology and psychiatry).

**Dr. Leyla: What is reintegration and why is it important?**
Dr. Rush: In many cultures, especially tribal groups, when an individual is ill, the whole cultures is sick and curing occurs in a communal setting with sickness representing "outside." Social reintegration is part of the process of wellness that is bringing the person from "outside" (sick, possessed by demons, taboo violation) to "inside" or bringing the individual and system back into balance. In Western culture, sickness and treatment are individual issues and not perceived as "culture out of balance." We don't provide rituals to signal cure or reintegrate the individual back to his group. This is especially notable when there is a psychiatric diagnosis which in itself represents a stigma, and the individual is often ignored or placed in special "homes" (halfway houses) often making reintegration to a "normal" life impossible.

**Dr. Leyla: If Western medicine is more concerned about illness maintenance than treating the cause, why is it the standard healthcare in our society?**
Dr. Rush: Western medicine has been the gold standard in our society since the late 19th Century. After 1912, with lack of funding for other medical practices (homeopathic, naturopathic, eclectic), allopathic medicine became the only game in town, a monopoly. This is why it is the standard in the US. The American Medical Association AMA has passed laws that will prevent a change in this standard any time soon.[7]

**Dr. Leyla: What kind of laws?**
Dr. Rush: The medical profession seems to operate on the assumption that they are a different type of business, one that has to be standardized under the name of science. This has allowed the AMA to create a political monopoly. However, without standardization you can't conduct clinical research, which we need.

**Dr. Leyla: Why do you believe that patients continue to go to medical doctors?**
Dr. Rush: The reason for this is visibility through advertisements, news updates on promising therapies, and of course various TV shows. When herbal medicines are reposted in the news, rarely do the news programmers contact an herbalist or someone who uses herbs in medicine.

Instead, they call in a medical doctor, and most know very little about alternative forms of medicine. In fact, they are constrained by the AMA from practicing alternative therapies. Thus, the consumer doesn't think of other alternatives, or even know that there are options. More important, insurance companies recognize and pay for Western medical doctors, and going to a specialist in an alternative therapy usually requires out-of-pocket payment.

**Dr. Leyla: What other types of healthcare have you studied?**
Dr. Rush:
- Ayurvedic Medicine - The major teaching of Ayurvedic medicine is that the individual is not a collection of parts

but an integrated whole. The human body is also universe. This tradition takes into account the environment you live within (house, workplace, etc.), relationships with others, your job, diet, weather patterns, seasons of the year, and so on.

- Chinese Medicine - Most people in the US have heard of Chinese medicine and especially acupuncture, or the insertion of needles along meridian points to effect physiological changes in the body. The Chinese philosophy is more elaborate and sees the body, the world, and the universe as an interconnected whole.

- Naturopathic Medicine - Closely connected to Ayurvedic medicine of India and Nature Cure of Europe is naturopathic medicine. The main concentration of naturopathy is cause of illness rather than suppressing symptoms as in the case of Western biomedicine. According the naturopathic philosophy, most illness is caused by malnutrition and cellular toxicity rather than germs and bad genes.

- Western Medicine - In medical anthropology, Western medicine may be compared to taking your car to the shop for repair. Something isn't running smoothly so you take it to the repair shop for a diagnosis and for them to patch it up.

**Dr. Leyla: Is Western medicine superior for any aspects of healthcare? When should someone rely on a medical doctor and when should they go holistic?**
Dr. Rush: Yes, Western biomedicine is superior in many ways, especially in terms of surgical procedures. Genetic engineering, as another example, shows promise for dealing with diabetes (and many other conditions); slowing aging, and tissue regeneration.

In terms of everyday health, other traditions (mentioned above) concentrate on diet, detox, and prevention in general. Prevention, curiously enough, hasn't been a strong point for Western biomedicine perhaps because healthy people don't need doctors.

But individual health is only part of the equation since individual health is directly related to social health. In our own time we see many more somatic complaints, inability to sleep, higher divorce rates, higher drug use and abuse, high unemployment, a divisive political regime, and so on. Social health and its causes and correction are not the domain of the medical establishment. Even most psychiatrists pay little attention to the larger picture and usually prescribe drugs.

**Dr. Leyla: What steps do you recommend to someone who has gone to a medical doctor and would like to switch to alternative or natural treatments?**
Dr. Rush: The first thing is your own personal diagnosis—what are your symptoms, how long have you had them, what in your life could be related to these symptoms?

Next, make some appointments with qualified individuals—naturopath, acupuncturist, homeopath, etc., and find out what they have to offer. Any type of diagnosis requires some sort of verification and this is a problem as many traditions, i.e. Chinese or Ayurvedic Medicine use references and terms that are foreign to most. Because of this, I also suggest that the individual read up on a tradition so that terms and references sound less foreign.

All surgical procedures should be performed by a qualified surgeon. Always get, not only a second opinion, but a third opinion before any surgery is performed.

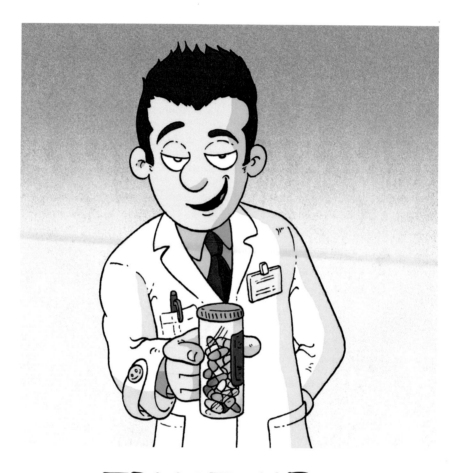

TRUST ME...
I`M A PHARMACIST

## CHAPTER 3

# DOCTORS AND PHARMACISTS

*Most doctors are prisoners of their education and shackled by their profession.* *~Richard Diaz*

## WHAT REALLY IS A DOCTOR?

Doctors and pharmacists start out on their individual journeys as eager students—energetic, intelligent, motivated—determined to face the academic challenges and financial risk of attending medical or pharmacy school. Their intentions are positive, including:

- Wanting to help people by improving patient health;
- Being awarded the prestigious title of *doctor* and being respected by society;
- Earning an income that affords a comfortable lifestyle; and
- Dreaming of making a difference, changing, and/or saving lives.

After spending years of time and energy, and often accumulating a significant amount of student loans, they are ready to hang that diploma on their office walls. That is when the reality sets in. These hope-filled individuals have buried themselves in a medical system that is not what it seems to be. Their ideals of becoming healthcare experts and helping people have devolved into the reality that they are slaves of pharmaceutical and insurance companies.

In fact, they've been sucker-punched into one of the biggest societal scams in our country: the American healthcare system.

Take a moment to consider these disturbing facts:

- Most medical doctors and pharmacists receive very little or no education regarding holistic health;
- Nutritional education is minimal at best;
- Cleansing the body of toxins is a non-standard medical procedure that is considered *alternative* in terms of health maintenance, and is only utilized for diagnostic procedures such as prior to an endoscope or colonoscopy; and
- Medical doctors have not been taught the strategic truth that human thoughts and feelings are directly linked to and can positively or negatively impact, our health.[36]

Today in America, doctors and pharmacists are not the healthcare providers we believe them to be, and often not the healthcare provider they expected to become.

Rather, they are educated by pharmaceutical companies and have become experts in administering drugs—as human tools in the drug companies' toolboxes. They are practitioners of a business methodology that needs patients in order to succeed. In exchange, they are highly paid and granted impressive titles with automatic respect. To be blunt, whether they know it or not, they are selling their souls and integrity, to pharmaceutical companies.[37]

Yet, on the other hand, there are areas in healthcare where medical doctors are indisputably more effective than alternative or natural treatments.

Medical doctors have the most sophisticated technology to diagnose a patient's condition, including MRIs and CAT scans. Additionally, for car accidents, broken bones or surgeries, doctors cannot be replaced by alternative means. Also, there are some drugs that have saved people's lives.

The problem occurs when doctors overstep their boundaries. They do not understand their own limitations, and often disregard the strengths of alternative methods. In fact, a doctor can diagnose a condition as *incurable*, or pain as *untreatable*. The doctors speak of a condition being *incurable* as if they are the all-knowing, final answer to one's health—as if there are no other options available. In fact, doctors will consider a condition *terminal* rather than learn about the other choices available. And, much of society trusts them and depends upon them for all their healthcare needs.

The reality is that there are numerous patients who have been cured of doctor-defined *incurable* conditions by alternative and natural remedies.[38] In fact, I have included several interviews in this book with people who have suffered for years after depending on the medical system, and regained their health through alternative and holistic means.

In later chapters I share their stories so others can see the possibilities that exist.

Please note I am not labeling doctors and pharmacists as *bad* or *evil*. My point is that having the title *doctor* is not really enough to earn unquestionable authority and respect. Modern doctors are not trained in total healthcare, nor are they trained in what is possible in the world. They are only trained in what is possible with drugs and surgery as a response to any illness.

And, the general population is programmed to trust and believe their doctor as the authority figure. At issue is that these messages are ingrained in us, both subliminally and blatantly. We listen to our doctor, we watch the drug commercials on television, and then we demand our pills—making us part of the problem.[39]

## THE MOST TRUSTED PROFESSION

When I was in pharmacy school, the instructors consistently promoted that, year after year, pharmacists rank high on the list of *most trusted professions*. This farce remains in existence.

Here is an excerpt from a recent article in *Pharmacy Times*:

Among respondents, 73 percent rated the honesty and ethical

standards of pharmacists as "very high" or "high," according to the survey, which measures the public's trust of professionals across diverse disciplines, including but not limited to healthcare.[40]"

These polls always make me wonder, who is conducting them and who is responding? This is another example of how the message is ingrained in our minds.

## ABUSE OF DOCTOR TITLE

I've been a pharmacist now for over 12 years. With that I have earned the title *doctor*, which I use when I want to establish myself as credible. And with that, I have seen how people respond to my title and the automatic trust and respect afforded me.[41]

But the drug companies have also caught on to this. In fact, they hire professionals that are *doctors* with the only goal to use their name on a study, to establish more credibility. And these doctors don't even have to do the work; the studies are written by ghostwriters! The drug companies have noticed the credibility and power that comes with the doctor title, and have learned how to use that knowledge to profit. For example:

He was abusing his doctor title. It was misleading to have the title *doctor* on a card about anti-aging, as many would assume that he is a medical doctor, or at least a type of doctor that would be related to his business.

However, there are no regulations against it.

In my opinion, the title doctor is completely overrated in our society. If someone has the title doctor, it doesn't mean that they are the complete authority.[42]

## QUALITY OF DOCTORS

There's an old joke that goes like this:
Q: What do you call the medical student that graduates last in his class?

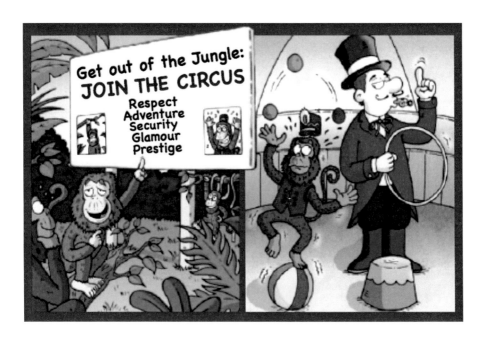

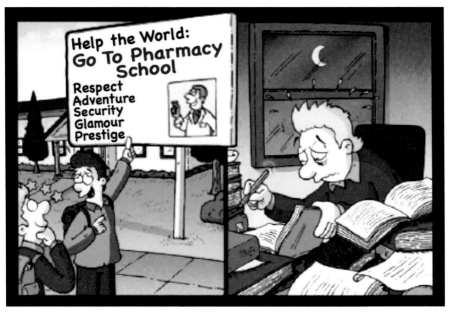

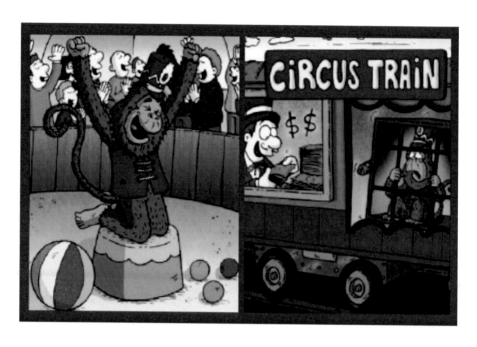

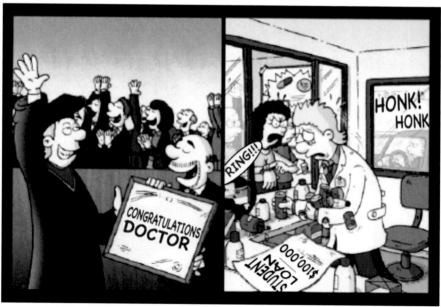

A:   A doctor.

Not all doctors are created equal.  As with any profession, the knowledge and quality of doctors can vary greatly.

Here are two examples of this phenomenon, based on my own experiences:

### Example 1 - a good doctor:

While attending pharmacy school I became really sick with a chest cold.  Not to be too graphic, but I was coughing up green stuff from my lungs like I'd never seen before.  I decided that I definitely needed an antibiotic.  And since I was a student of pharmacy, I was excited that I could intelligently discuss the pill regimen with my doctor.  I envisioned we would discuss whether it was gram positive, or gram negative, which bacteria was likely causing the problem, and which drug would be the best choice.  I went to the campus physician and he examined me and asked the usual questions.

His suggested treatment: Ibuprofen every four to six hours, around the clock, so I could feel better while my body healed itself.  I sat there, angry and annoyed.  He called me on it, catching me off-guard:

Doctor:   *"You look upset, what's wrong?"*
Patient:   *"I – I was expecting an antibiotic, its green!"*
Doctor:   *"You can't tell what the cause is by the color, and if it's a virus, an antibiotic won't do anything but mess up the normal bacteria in your stomach.  You don't need an antibiotic; your body can fight it off."*
Patient:   *"Huh, okay."*

I didn't fully understand the significance of his viewpoint until much later.  I realized that my expectations, reflective of the norm, were a huge source of the problem.  I was upset because I went to a doctor's appointment and came away empty handed—no prescription to fill.  I felt cheated.  Why even go to the doctor?  The doctor explained that we do so for their knowledge and expertise, not to get a pill.

Needless to say, he was right.

My body fought off the infection; I'm still alive and well. Of great importance, I gave my immune system the opportunity to work its natural processes; I have yet to experience a sickness like that since.

The fact is the human body needs two weeks to build the right antibodies that will fight off a specific infection. After these natural agents are created, the next time the body is exposed to a similar affliction, the antibodies are already created and they are therefore prepared to fight with only a few days needed to recover. Rest is what the body often needs in time of illness.

However, with our fast-paced society, and insurance companies willing to pay, many demand an antibiotic for a quick recovery at a low price. In my case, I actually felt as if I *deserved* an antibiotic. From my perspective this was normal, it was expected and I had no idea of the problems that taking one could cause.

But every time we take an antibiotic, we are interrupting our bodies' natural response to build antibodies to handle the infection naturally. When another infection comes along, the body will not be prepared and once again will depend on an antibiotic to fight infections. This overuse of antibiotics is what has led to the problem of resistance, where stronger and stronger antibiotics are needed and eventually may not work at all.[43]

### Example 2 - bad doctor:
My friend's 15 year-old son was morbidly obese. Hoping to find him some help, she made an appointment with a psychologist who was covered under her HMO. This appointment consisted of a four minute consultation/conversation, whereby two prescriptions were given: Wellbutrin, an antidepressant, and phentermine, an appetite suppressant and stimulant—basically a legalized form of speed.

My friend called me for my opinion. "Should I fill it?"

I emphatically said no and explained that phentermine may help lose weight, temporarily, but side effects include edginess and irritability. Since the drug is recommended for limited timeframes (remember, it's SPEED), once he stops taking it he will probably regain the weight, possibly more than he initially lost. Additionally, both Wellbutrin and phentermine cause insomnia, so he may have trouble sleeping. Sarcastically speaking, on the good side, the antidepressant will at least make him feel happy while this doctor is screwing everything else up.

So what is going on here? Consider these questions:

1. Was the doctor just lazy, going through the motions?
2. Was she giving the patient (and mom) what they wanted— a prescription to solve the problem?
3. Did she automatically prescribe a medication that fell within coverage guidelines, thus minimizing any potential hassle (for both herself and the patient) with the insurance company?
4. Was this practitioner desirous of providing a better, more informed treatment, but simply tired of fighting the fight?
5. Or, does this practitioner have any knowledge at all of other possibilities for treatment of obesity, besides medications?

In my friend's situation, it is unclear whether the problem lay with the doctor, insurance company policy and procedure, or (misinformed) demands from the patient. As evidenced by this example, sadly, the young man's good health was **NOT** the priority.

I hope the above examples shed some light on our current health crisis. It is unfortunate that my doctor's prescribed regimen (Example 1) is not the norm. At the same time, there are others like him, who can provide exceptional service based on knowledge of many forms of healing or wellness maintenance.

His method, to educate rather than automatically prescribe, regardless of the resistances and struggles caused by the patient's desires, is the best way to practice medicine.

## FINDING A GOOD DOCTOR

In seeking quality guidance from a doctor, here is a list of suggested questions to help the reader discover a physician's methodology. In this way, you have a degree of control. Ask them:

- Do you believe in holistic medicine? Or, do you view these holistic providers as quacks?
- What do you think is the role of holistic medicine in today's society?
- Are you open to other forms of healthcare?
- Where do you think patients can find the best solutions, for maintaining wellness and dealing with sickness? Where is (are) their best resource(s)?
- What do you think about cleansing?
- Some folks in the holistic medicine realm claim that 99 percent of diseases are caused by what we eat. What are your thoughts on this?

Questions like these may help you decide if the doctor is open to other forms of healthcare, and whether he has knowledge and awareness beyond standard solutions. The physician may not have expertise in *all methods* of wellness and sick care, but it's also important that he wields a good understanding of American medicine's limitations, as well as being open to the other options that are available.

Communicating with your doctor to understand his or her perspective is the key. These questions will help you find out if your potential provider is a slave to the business model of drug companies, or if your doctor is a free thinker, with the best of intentions.[44]

## AND THE PATIENTS

Patients must stop expecting a prescription to fix all their ailments. They must understand that drugs are only one option, one piece of the puzzle, and usually not the best choice.

**34**

As patients, we have a duty to understand our own bodies and health, and take a more active role, rather than just listening to our doctors and filling a prescription.

## THE FUTURE

Americans are in a rut. There are not enough people *really* thinking, or taking the time to analyze the deep-seeded problems in our healthcare system. Instead, the formula for wellness has been defined for us, and stamped into our individual and collective psyche. Any hint of physical or emotional pain is reconciled with the perfect pill, prescribed by a doctor or a television commercial, and paid for by health insurance.

Of even greater concern, doctors are unaware of a better solution, other than which pill to prescribe. And finally, even if they present a different option, oftentimes it's really not what many patients are looking for.

Let me restate, I do believe that doctors play an important role in our healthcare system.

However, it is important that they realize there is so much more to health and wellness than what was taught in medical school. As long as the patients are demanding their drugs, the doctors are writing the prescriptions, and the insurance companies are paying for the medications, then the pharmaceutical companies will continue to profit, whether the medication is good for you or not.

## POINTS TO REMEMBER:

- Although doctors and pharmacists are regarded as experts on health, the truth is that they are only trained in drugs.

- Neither medical schools nor pharmacy schools require their students to have training in or knowledge of the holistic view of health—body, mind, and spirit.

## INTERVIEW WITH AYURVEDIC PRACTITIONER DR. SIVA MOHAN

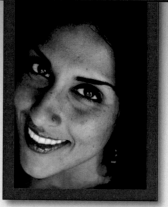

*As a child, Dr. Mohan had aspired to become a medical doctor. Her journey started with neuroscience, which sparked her interest in the mind-body connection. In medical school and during her Public Health Masters she focused her studies on the extension of the mind-body relationship—the effects of community, development and culture on health behavior.*

*After a year of working in clinical health, Dr. Mohan came to the realization that the work involved symptom alleviation rather than curing, or healing. The work also rarely took people's lifestyles into consideration.*

*Dr. Mohan believes that lifestyles and habits determine our health. This, along with her cultural heritage, led her to leave the medical profession and study Ayurveda.*

*Dr. Mohan now practices Ayurveda and yoga, and is able to address health with a personal, individualized, and holistic approach. Her professional goals continue to be writing, lecturing, and spreading the awareness of Ayurveda and how it can complement modern medicine.*

**Dr. Leyla: Where did you go to medical school?**
Dr. Mohan: Cornell University.

**Dr. Leyla: Why did you go to medical school?**
Dr. Mohan: I had just spent four years at Pomona College learning about the mind-body interface, with more focus on the brain and mind. It was natural to then spend time learning about how the body works. Plus, I was one of those kids that said they wanted to be a doctor

—at age 5. I don't know why, yet the drive was so strong that I never questioned it.

**Dr. Leyla: What were your ideas about medicine when you went to medical school?**
Dr. Mohan: In my second year, when we began heavy clinical work, I quickly became disillusioned with what was considered *healing*. I realized what we were actually doing was symptom palliation and very rarely *curing* anything. Some look at surgery as a cure because it means the problem is completely gone; that's not what I'm talking about. Why do you have this problem that requires surgery in the first place? Addressing that and resolving the underlying problem is what a cure means to me.

Also, I grew up in a family where we rarely took medicines; seeing the extent to which the medical industrial complex is intertwined with the pharmaceutical industry was saddening. Even on a systems level, I saw how health policies made on a population level aren't necessarily best for people on an individual level. This, in my opinion, is the big catch-22 of public health and of Western medicine; there have to be standards for safety and accountability, but that takes away the art and personalization of evaluation and treatment.

**Dr. Leyla: Can you give an example?**
Dr. Mohan: Sure. Recently I was consulting on a public health program in India. In some developing countries, it makes sense to insert an IUD for birth control right after a woman delivers a baby. This is because oral contraception is not always socially acceptable and getting the women back into the clinic several weeks later for IUD placement is unlikely. It can be a great ordeal to get to the clinic for many of the women who live in rural areas.

Many of the women desire contraception, so they can have the IUD inserted after delivery to address two issues in one visit. However, right after giving birth is not necessarily the best time to have an IUD inserted. It can lead to further problems and infections. On a population level, this reproductive initiative makes sense. As a woman who has home-birthed my children, the idea of having an IUD inserted into my uterus right after delivery is completely counter-intuitive, both physically and emotionally.

**Dr. Leyla: Why did you continue with Ayurveda?**
Dr. Mohan: When I made the decision to not practice Western medicine, I had a bit of a midlife crisis.

Here I had spent my whole life thinking I was going to be a doctor, so not practicing medicine was a big shift. I considered moving to some remote part of the world where I could be a *real* doctor practicing in the bush, making a significant difference in people's health. But even that is an allopathic model in which the patient gives over the power to heal him/herself to the doctor.

I believe that our lifestyles and habits determine our health, and this means we have the power to heal ourselves. By this point in my life, I was too drawn to the concept of healing being an empowerment process, and this, along with my cultural heritage, drew me to Ayurveda.

It was not an easy decision to return to school having already completed two postgraduate degrees. In the end, I knew I had to study Ayurveda because I wanted to apply it in my own life, and with my own children.

**Dr. Leyla: How do you treat people with Ayurvedic medicine?**
Dr. Mohan: I don't treat people, they treat themselves. I just educate them on how to do that. I map out how the various facets of their lives are playing into their health patterns: physically and mentally.

**Dr. Leyla: What does Ayurvedic medicine involve?**
Dr. Mohan: At its core, Ayurveda means getting in touch with your spirit, or inner voice—and listening to it—when you make decisions. In my work with clients, we use changes in lifestyle, routine, diet, job, relationship dynamics, yoga, meditation, herbal formulas—anything is game—to help them find a way of living that is healthiest for them. You see, in Ayurveda, we are all unique, so each person's healthiest lifestyle/diet/habits, etc. will also be unique to them.

There are so many alternative therapies and natural care options these days that people are overwhelmed. My role is to help them figure out what is best for them through the consistent language and platform of Ayurveda. We do this over and over again in many areas of their lives until they can do it for themselves and are no longer dependent on me.

**Dr. Leyla: What does a typical Ayurvedic appointment consist of?**
Dr. Mohan: Initially I'll sit with them for two hours to learn the various *energy* inputs in their lives: How they are managing their job's stresses, kids, relationships, finances, diet, and exercise?

From this I get a sense of the patterns, and combine that information with a pulse and tongue reading, to do a full analysis of their constitution, what imbalances are present and what specific issues need to be addressed in our sessions. From this I create a treatment plan outline.

By age 30, almost everyone has certain health patterns and becoming aware of them is quite empowering.

My treatment plans start with one system of the body and move forward by system (e.g., digestive first, then nervous system). Within a given system there may be several issues. For example, perhaps they have a low appetite, weight gain, gas, and bloating or slight nausea in the mornings. We will start addressing each of these issues before moving on to the next system.

How we specifically choose to address any given issue depends on each client—it could be a yoga pose, an herbal formula, a breath exercise, a diet change, and so on. I give out *homework* to really incorporate these assignments into their lives in between follow-up appointments. Follow-up appointments occur every two to three weeks.

I believe that long-term change happens slowly and requires ongoing support. So my process with my clients lasts between six months and two years. We proceed at the pace their life is taking them; one that will allow them to make sustainable changes. My process ends when they are comfortable with mapping for themselves which aspects of their lives are causing certain issues in the mind/emotions and the body, and adjust accordingly with the tools they've learned. At that point, they may come to see me as they need to, but they are in a new state of awareness, and thus empowered to own their health.

**Dr. Leyla: Do you also use your medical knowledge/background?**
Dr. Mohan: Every day, I use the incredible knowledge I learned in Western medicine. Most people walk in with a few diagnoses, or health issues (e.g., migraines, irregular period, chronic low back pain, anxiety, recurrent sinusitis, and the list goes on). Understanding how the body works allows me to educate them on what they are experiencing and how they are being treated in a Western context. It also enables me to understand how our process will interface with their Western care and how integration can best take place.

Oftentimes, clients wish to decrease their pharmaceutical load—I help educate them on how to interact with their doctors to achieve their desired results. Most of the doctors are surprised to see how the patients have healed themselves. I've had incredible stories: clients ovulating after 15 years of unsuccessful fertility treatments and completely healing ulcerative colitis without medication, are a few that come to mind.

**Dr. Leyla: What are the advantages and disadvantages of Ayurvedic medicine?**
Dr. Mohan: The Ayurvedic approach of addressing the root cause of disease—our lifestyles and our habits—is the strongest form of prevention. However, through natural approaches, patients must be willing to change the energies in their lives and that means changing their lives.

If I'm going to tell you it is *your* lifestyle and habits that are manifesting in *your* body and in *your* mind, it is *your* lifestyle and habits that cause disease that puts lots of responsibility on you, the patient. This is a big shift from handing that responsibility over to medical professionals.

In Western medicine, a doctor gives me medicine and I can think I'm solving my problem by taking a pill. More and more these days, people are becoming weary of taking a pill. They are questioning the side effects, paying more attention to how they feel with the medication, and becoming more unwilling to be dependent on a pill to feel good.

The great advantage of Ayurveda, is that it cultivates a new level of awareness. Once you go through this process, you can draw on it for the rest of your life, in any health situation.

**Dr. Leyla: Does Ayurvedic medicine have any limitations?**
Dr. Mohan: Again, you must make some changes in your life and habits. Other limitations of the practice of Ayurveda today include inconsistency in how it is practiced. Many practitioners operate as though it is just a natural healing option—just take herbs instead of medicines. For me, it's deeper than that.

**Dr. Leyla: What are some common problems you see with Western medicine patients?**
Dr. Mohan: Because of pressures to maintain standards of care and the scare of malpractice lawsuits, medical care is over-standardized. Doctors must treat everyone the same, which ensures a lot of unnecessary diagnostic tests and prescriptions.

In the long run, this means increasing insurance prices, greater environmental waste, over-medication, and patients that are more estranged from their health process. Doctors are less empowered, as this automation of doctoring is taking the art out of the profession.

People have diseases yet they have no understanding of what the disease is, or the prognosis, or the medications. They are not encouraged to ask "how can I heal myself?" Doctors don't have time to explain, and they are not taught this approach in medical schools. There are many ways in which Western medicine is incredible and unparalleled. For chronic issues and prevention, it is a weak approach in my opinion.

**Dr. Siva Mohan**
**444 W. Ocean Blvd, Suite 800, Long Beach, CA 90802**
**(562) 986-1700**

**Svasthahealth.com**

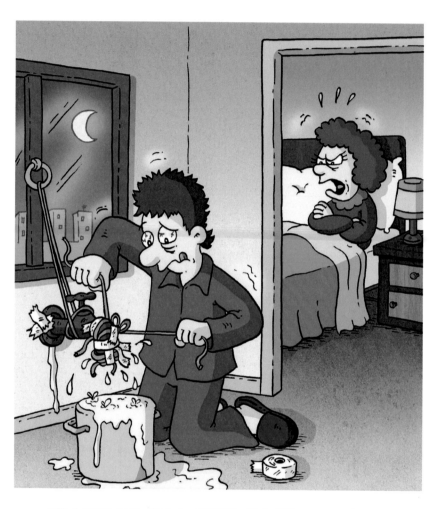

**JUST TURN OFF THE MAIN WATER LINE, DAMMIT!**

CHAPTER 4

# WHAT'S WRONG WITH AMERICAN MEDICINE?

*It is easy to get a thousand prescriptions but hard to get one single remedy.*
*~Chinese proverb*

What is American medicine's perspective on health? How do our trained physicians handle sicknesses? Most people have been to a doctor for an ailment of some sort. Most know the routine of waiting for a doctor, a quick examination, and leaving with a prescription. This is standard operating procedure.

Arthritis runs in my family: my grandmother, mother, and aunt all had problems with swelling in their joints. But, I was never worried because I knew that our country had good medical care available and there were several types of drugs on hand to treat it. I felt comfortable, that is, until I went to pharmacy school and really understood how doctors and drugs were handling medical conditions such as this.

## MAINTAINING BALANCE

It is important to understand that the human body is constantly striving to *manage* all its functions, from the simple to the amazingly complex.

For example, our bodies have several mechanisms in place to keep us alive—the heart for blood flow and the lungs for oxygen intake. In order for these and many other aspects of the body's health to operate properly, certain factors must be present and maintained in balance, including fluids, red blood cells, glucose, pH, electrolytes, and temperature, to name a few. This balancing act is essential for our bodies to survive and remain healthy.[45]

It is not unusual for most people to have experienced a fever or a swollen ankle in their lifetimes. In these instances, the body is sending out a vital sign that something is amiss, and it is working to regain balance and normal function. Often this is accompanied by pain that is being *broadcast* to the brain via the nervous system. This chapter provides an overview of the body's natural processes to regain balance. Examples will include tempature control, swelling and inflammation, diabetes, and infections.

## TEMPERATURE

The body maintains a temperature of 98.6°, with a normal range of 97.5°F to 98.9°F. When the body is overheated, we sweat to cool it down. Likewise when we are too cold, the body will shiver to create heat. Interestingly, the human body can only function normally in a narrow range of internal temperatures. Therefore shivering and perspiration are the body's response to keep the tempature within this range.[46]

When certain bacteria or viruses enter the body, one defense mechanism that the body uses is to raise its temperature—a fever—in order to create an environment in which the invader(s) cannot survive.

Although a fever is uncomfortable it does serve a very important purpose. Unfortunately, American society is inundated with advertisements for fever reducers, in order to bring comfort to the patient. But by so doing, these medications, primarily over-the-counter, can possibly assist in the survival of the body's invader, which will prolong the duration of the illness. Obviously, there are instances where an excessive fever is dangerous and needs to be professionally addressed. At this point a fever reducer should be taken. But the main point is that when the fever reducer is taken, it is actually making the patient more comfortable, in exchange for disrupting the body's natural response to an infection.[47]

Suppose that body shivers in response to cold are considered uncomfortable, painful, or inconvenient. The standard response by pharmaceutical companies would be to create a pill that stops the body from the *uncontrollable or chronic shaking* so the patient is more comfortable.

Again, this would only solve the symptom by stunting the body's response—and actually hinder the body's response to regain balance. The temperature would continue to drop, potentially creating future problems for other bodily functions.


## SWELLING AND INFLAMMATION

Similarly, swelling is the immune system's natural response to a physical injury, such as an ankle sprain.[48] In very simple terms, the blood vessels enlarge and allow the immune system to *repair* the affected area by clearing away all the torn tissue, and then bringing in proteins to rebuild and repair the damaged tissue.

The medical response to an ankle sprain is to reduce swelling by elevating the leg to reduce blood flow, applying ice, and taking an anti-inflammatory such as ibuprofen or naproxen. Although swelling is a natural response of the body to heal itself, the swelling can become excessive and painful. In this case, the decision to take steps to reduce swelling is appropriate as it allows the patient to be more comfortable and the body is still able to repair itself.

The situation is different, however, when chronic swelling occurs. There are several conditions that cause the body to swell on a long-term or chronic basis. Examples include: rheumatoid arthritis, asthma, ulcerative colitis, dermatitis, and allergic conditions such as rhinitis. These swelling diseases are typically addressed by focusing on patient comfort.

However, reducing swelling on a long term basis does not address the cause of the problem, which, in turn, allows the condition to progress. The pharmaceutical approach to handling this, in my opinion, is one of the biggest problems in American medicine. Many drugs will suppress symptoms rather than discover and respond to the cause.

If there is an underlying issue that symptoms are trying to bring to light, suppression of these signals is a bad approach. Once a symptom is suppressed, the condition will continue to brew under the surface, increasing the chances of an illness getting worse.[49] Additionally, the body often finds other ways to express the problem, which only leads to additional medications. In certain instances, extreme swelling may require medication, but all too often a doctor will prescribe a pill to address a patient's discomfort. So, temporary relief may come at the expense of allowing the body to naturally repair itself, or at least slowing down the healing process.

In cases of a swollen ankle or fever, the body can often heal itself despite the suppression of symptoms. However, with chronic illnesses, this approach can lead to additional problems, including the disease progressing, the body no longer responding to the medication, and long-term side effects. Then pill upon pill is prescribed. And since the original problem is never addressed or solved, the result is that Americans have become long term customers of doctors and drugs, and overly dependent on external solutions to relieve symptoms rather than the miracle of time and the body's internal mechanisms.[50]

## RHEUMATOID ARTHRITIS

Rheumatoid arthritis is a chronic condition that leads to inflammation of the joints and surrounding tissues. According to Western medicine, the cause is unknown and it is considered to be an autoimmune disease wherein the body's immune system attacks itself.[51]

Swelling of the joints is a warning sign; the body is responding to an imbalance—something is not right—and it is naturally attempting to correct itself. Let's take a look at American medicine's typical response to this condition.

A patient visits the doctor complaining about swelling of the joints. The doctor asks questions and exams the patient, and then sends him or her off to visit the pharmacy, script in hand.

*First Line Treatment*

The first treatment is usually an over-the-counter anti-inflammatory medication, such as aspirin or ibuprofen. These pills relieve the swelling and the patient's joints will feel better quickly. However, the underlying cause of the pain has not been addressed and will remain with the body.

The pain is suppressed yet the condition continues. Over time as the disease progresses, the initial medication will be insufficient and the dose must be increased. If the patient continues on a high dose of ibuprofen (800mg/3X daily), excess acid in the stomach is created, causing a debilitating side effect to the stomach lining. The protective barriers of the stomach may then erode, leading to an ulcer. (Note the cause of patient's joint inflammation remains embedded.)

Now, of course, the ulcer must be treated—with prescription medications. The dosage of the anti-inflammatory must be decreased or discontinued altogether. So what's the next step?

*Second Line Treatment*

The second line treatment occurs when the patient is no longer comfortable, and is either not responding properly to the initial treatment, or is experiencing residual side effects that are creating more problems to address. Keep in mind that swelling is a normal function of the immune system.

Once again, according to Western medicine the cause is unknown. Treatments consist of reducing swelling however possible using different, stronger medications. Here are some options for the doctor to consider when the first treatment is no longer effective:

- Continue the anti-inflammatory and add another medication that protects the stomach (Misoprostol). The side effect of this treatment plan—lots of diarrhea.
- Switch the patient to another anti-inflammatory in the same class, which will delay but eventually progress to the same problems.
- Add a glucosamine supplement.

Again, if an ulcer occurs, the patient must stop taking anti-inflammatory medication, and use the next option.

### Third Line Treatment

The next line of treatment includes disease-modifying anti-rheumatic drugs (DMARDs), which are said to slow the progression of the disease. The drugs include methotrexate, gold salts, and hydroxychloroquine. However, there are some severe and debilitating side effects that come with these.

### Fourth Line Treatment

Lastly, prednisone—a synthetic immunosuppressant—will be prescribed. Yes, the standard response to medically dealing with rheumatoid arthritis is to *suppress* the workings of the immune system by introducing a steroid regimen. Because the immune system is the source of the swelling, the *logic* is to block this swelling function in order to minimize the discomfort of the condition.

The insanity is that a suppressed immune system exposes the body to all kinds of infections and other diseases. Thus, chances are that our medical industry has created another customer for life, yet still hasn't treated the original problem.

And on a side note, the risks inherent to steroid use are well documented. The short-term side effects are manageable, like stomach upset and fluid retention. Long-term, though, these synthetic drugs cause a bundle of problems. Some of these include osteoporosis, thinning of the skin, depression, diabetes, joint and muscle pain, increased eye pressure, puffing of the face, bruising, weight gain, and tiredness. Keep in mind these are all in addition to the increased vulnerability to infections, cancer and other diseases caused by the suppression of the immune system.

I like to compare standard medical practice as it pertains to the human body with an image of a beautiful, stately mansion that has a leaky bathroom faucet. Obviously, that annoying dripping sound is affecting your peace of mind, so you contact the *specialist* plumber who suggests plumbing tape to patch the leak.

The silence returns, and you sleep well. At some point, though, the tape wears down and the leak is back with a vengeance, and is getting worse. So you go back to that specialist, who recommends a different kind of tape, which is stronger and lasts longer. Over time this tape also wears down and the leaks then sprout in different spots. The drip returns. You return to the specialist who now recommends that you shut off your water.

The problem is fixed—there is no more leaking! But at what cost? Now there is no water in the household, which is inconvenient, but the leak is gone! You can buy water and actually get by. But then again, if there's a fire or other emergency, there will be big problems.

Similarly, in rheumatoid arthritis the swelling is caused by the immune system response, or overreaction. If you reduce the function of the immune system, the inconvenience caused by the swelling is solved. However, the price you pay for this is some severe side effects as well as a suppressed immune system. Even if you are completely healthy otherwise, if you come across a bacterial or viral challenge, your immune system will not be prepared to fight that fire.[52]

## DIABETES

Epidemic proportions of American citizens are directly and indirectly affected by diabetes. Beyond the obvious health risks, there are some statistics that are truly disturbing:

- Nearly 25.8 million people have one form of diabetes, and it is estimated that an additional seven million have type 2 diabetes and do not realize it.[53]
- Approximately 90-95 percent of individuals with diabetes have type 2 diabetes.[54]
- Type 2 diabetes is directly related to diet and lifestyle; prevention starts with human choice and habit.
- Both types of this disease generate huge revenue streams for drug manufacturers.

## Digestion

To better understand diabetes, let us follow the flow of food in a healthy body. First, we chew and swallow our food. In the stomach the food is digested and then absorbed into the bloodstream. The liver enzymes break it down, separating valuable nutrients from waste. The carbohydrates are broken down into glucose (source of energy).

This glucose travels through the bloodstream and is delivered to the variety of cells that make up our bodies. The glucose enters the cells, and the cells convert the glucose to energy.

However, in order for the glucose to enter the cells, insulin, the *doorman*, must be present. Otherwise the glucose cannot enter and be utilized.

In a normal and balanced world the right amount of sugar is consumed and the insulin helps get the glucose into the cells to become energy.

## Types of Diabetes

The two types of diabetes:

Type 1 – is considered an autoimmune disease and occurs when the pancreas can no longer create *insulin*. The standard treatment is to provide replacement insulin.

Type 2 – was formerly known as adult-onset diabetes, but is now found in teenagers, and the trend is creeping towards younger children. Despite the presence of insulin, the body's cells develop *insulin resistance* in which the glucose cannot enter the cells.

The main distinction between type 1 and type 2 diabetes is *lack of insulin* versus *insulin resistance*. However, both lead to an excess of glucose in the bloodstream.[55]

Type 2 diabetes is associated with excessive sugar (glucose) intake and obesity. At some point, the cells no longer want or need any more glucose.

As a result the insulin that normally carries the sugar into the cells does not work as efficiently. This is referred to as *insulin resistance*. This is the beginning of the imbalance—there is too much glucose in the bloodstream.

It is this excess of glucose in the bloodstream that causes the imbalance and leads to the symptoms of diabetes.

The bloodstream however, works to maintain certain concentrations of glucose, nutrients, proteins, etc. Otherwise the blood will become too thick and inefficient. To compensate, the body pulls water out of the cells and into the bloodstream. The result is what causes the most well-known symptoms of diabetes: thirst and increased urination.

- Thirst is caused when the fluid is pulled from cells and transferred to bloodstream to compensate for increased glucose in blood.
- Increased urination occurs as the body works to eliminate the excess fluid in the bloodstream.

## Treatments

*Type 1 Diabetes*
Treatment for type 1 diabetes is simple since there is no insulin being created, hence insulin injections must be administered.

*Type 2 Diabetes*
The treatment for type 2 diabetes begins with a significant shift in diet, along with improvements to lifestyle, as well as establishing a consistent exercise routine. The appropriate adjustments are dependent upon a person's abilities and willingness to change.

The next option for type 2 diabetes is medication as there are several drugs to choose from. Here is a brief overview of a few of the commonly prescribed medications.

- **Metformin (Glucophage)** decreases the amount of glucose produced in liver, decreases the intestinal absorption of glucose, and improves insulin sensitivity.[56]

**51**

Translation: less glucose is produced by the liver and absorbed in the stomach. The third function, *improves insulin sensitivity,* means that even though the cells are rejecting the glucose, this medication will work to override the rejection and *force* glucose into the cell.

- **Thiazolidinediones (Avandia, Actos)** decreases insulin resistance in the periphery and in the liver, resulting in increased insulin-dependent glucose disposal and a decrease in glucose production by the liver.

Translation: again, the glucose is not being readily absorbed by the cells, so the drug will push the cells to better absorb the glucose. On a side note, one medication in this class, Avandia, has been pulled off the market after it was found to cause a 43 percent increase in the risk of a heart attack. Also, there is now a warning that Actos can "cause or exacerbate congestive heart failure."[57]

- **Sulfonylurea (Glipizide, Glyburide)** decreases blood glucose by stimulating insulin release from the pancreas and thereby increasing tissue sensitivity to insulin.[58]

Translation: it causes more insulin to circulate in the blood, and also increases insulin sensitivity to get more glucose into the cells and out of the bloodstream.

All of these medications will attempt to *increase insulin sensitivity,* which in essence means even though the cells do not want any more glucose the medications are attempting to jam it in there anyway.

The "experts" from WebMD.com and the American Diabetes Association describes insulin resistance as "when the body does not respond appropriately to insulin".[59] This implies that the body is defective and not functioning properly. *However, this is not true.*

**The body is in fact overwhelmed with glucose from eating excess sugar and processed foods.**

This is what causes the insulin resistance. As an analogy, your trash can is filled to the rim and you keep putting trash in it, so it overflows and trash falls on the ground. Is your trash can not working appropriately? Or has it reached capacity and is overwhelmed?

Insulin resistance is not a defect in the body's function. Rather it is the body asking, if not begging you, to consume less glucose.

## Blood Tests

When patients test their blood glucose for diabetes, they are actually measuring the blood glucose levels. If a medication is effective, it will somehow decrease the level of glucose in the bloodstream, which will decrease the symptoms of thirst and increased urination. If the amount of glucose in the bloodstream is lowered, then the medication is considered effective.

However, the medications are working to get the glucose out of the blood to pass this test, they are not working to get to the root of the problem, or to regain balance. Rather, they cure a symptom and creates a long-term customer. To regain balance, there has to be much less glucose consumed. In fact, many diabetics have recovered completely from changes in diet and exercise. For the more extreme souls, a natural and raw food diet can cure a diabetic in a matter of weeks.

Additionally, each of these diabetic medications have side effects, including: heart problems, hypoglycemia, dizziness, and weight gain. Therefore, many diabetics become fully reliant upon pills and the medical system, ultimately living a life of expanding health problems, debilitating side effects, and risks of poor drug interactions.

In fact, diabetic patients are one of insurance companies' biggest expenses, costing over $174 billion annually.[60] This is a frightening, unending, burdensome, and costly existence for approximately 10 percent of American society, especially when much simpler and natural solutions exist.

## ANTIBIOTICS

In 1940, penicillin was the first antibiotic available on the market. People were excited about this wonder drug. It was able to treat a variety of infections that were previously deadly, like diphtheria, gangrene, pneumonia, syphilis and tuberculosis.[61]   In addition, if someone got wounded, often they would die from infection. This was even more significant as, in the 1940s, people were going to war. Many wounded soldiers would have died from infections. Now penicillin could save them.[62]

But what's happened since then?  In one word: overuse.

### Problems

There are two big problems with taking antibiotics.

First, when you get exposed to bacteria, or an infection, your body's immune system kicks in and creates antibodies. Antibodies work to identify and neutralize foreign invaders such as bacteria and viruses. These antibodies are very specific for an individual disease-causing agent.

It takes two weeks for your body's immune system to build up the antibodies to fight off a specific infection.[63]  During that time a patient should slow down, rest, and drink fluids. By giving your body the time to heal, the antibodies have a chance to build up and make your immune system stronger. Then, if you're ever exposed to a similar invader in the future, it only takes a day or so to recover, as the army is already built so your immune system is now prepared.

When a patient takes a prescription antibiotic, the patient may recover more quickly. However, the body's immune response is interrupted. Therefore, if exposed to a similar infection in the future, the body will not be prepared and it will be more likely to be susceptible to the more resistant infections that are difficult to treat.

The second problem is that every time an antibiotic is taken, the medication isn't specific enough to kill only the bacteria causing the symptoms. There

**54**

are lots of good bacteria in the body that serve a purpose for digestion, balance and are necessary for good health. When an antibiotic is taken it also kills those as well, causing your system to be even more off balance.

Following the pattern of other drug treatments, antibiotics may do the job, but the patient will be more susceptible to problems and more severe infections in the future.

A big problem is that many patients want and expect antibiotics for simple colds and congestion. The fact is, the more you take antibiotics, the less prepared your immune system will be and the less able to fight off infections. Plus, because of the overuse of antibiotics and the ever evolving nature of bacteria, there are now resistant strains of bacteria that available antibiotics cannot treat.[64]

## A BETTER WAY

If your body can fight off an infection, let it. Especially for cough and colds in otherwise healthy patients who don't have complications. Allow your body to rest and recover on its own. Allow your immune system to build up and get stronger. Only take antibiotics as a last resort, or if the infection will lead to more serious problems.

## SUMMARY

Rheumatoid arthritis and diabetes are two common conditions in our society. Additionally, antibiotics have the pattern of a quick solution with potential long-term problems. Like myself before pharmacy school, I'm sure that many have faith in the drugs and medical system. But, I'm fairly certain that if they really come to understand how bad the treatment regimens are, many will search for alternatives.

Although these examples of rheumatoid arthritis, diabetes, and infections are specific, they demonstrate the pattern of "ease a symptom and create profit" that runs throughout much of the Western medicine treatment regimens.[65]

**POINTS TO REMEMBER:**

- The body has mechanisms to keep itself in balance.

- Suppressing these mechanisms does not treat the problem; it only hinders the warning sign.

- The idea behind much of American medicine is to suppress symptoms to make the patient feel more comfortable, and create a profit.

- Because American medicine rarely addresses the cause of conditions, patients often do not restore balance or regain health. Rather, they maintain an off-balance state, and in time require more and more drugs and medical treatment.

# HOLISTIC APPROACH TO HEALTH

Our bodies have several components that are necessary for the body to function properly. All these components must be kept in balance, and our body has mechanisms to maintain these components in balance.

For example, the body must maintain a certain temperature. If it gets too hot, the body sweats. When it's too cool, the body shivers.

Similarly, the body has mechanisms to keep all the other aspects in balance, including red blood cells, pH, glucose, fluids, bacteria, etc.

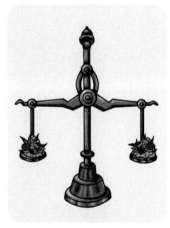

**1 - A Healthy Body**
*in balance*

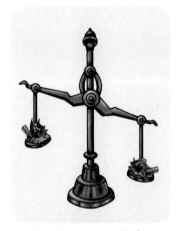

**2 - Patient is Sick**
*off balance*

**3 - Regain Balance**
A holistic practitioner will work to assist the patient to restore his or her body's balance, whether it's caused by nutrition, toxicity, emotions, etc.

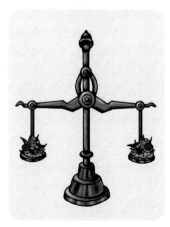

# WESTERN MEDICINE APPROACH TO HEALTH

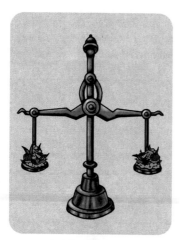

**1 - A Healthy Body**
*in balance*

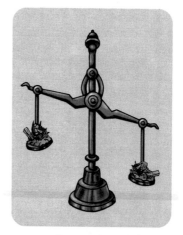

**2 - Patient is Sick**
*off balance*

**3 - Brace to Provide Relief**
In rheumatoid arthritis, a pill will be prescribed to reduce the swelling and make the patient more comfortable, but this does not address the cause.

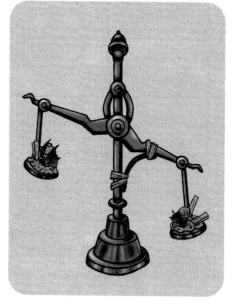

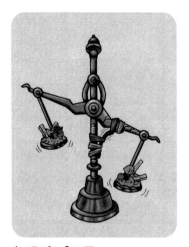

**4 - Relief is Temporary**
As the disease progresses and side effects occur.

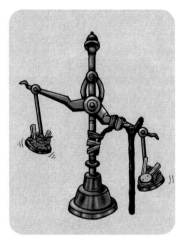

**5 - Another Brace**
Add another pill to ease the symptoms or relieve the side effects.

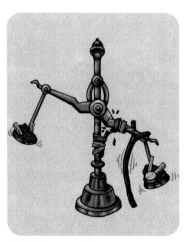

**6 - Disease Progresses**
Disease continues to progress and even more side effects occur.

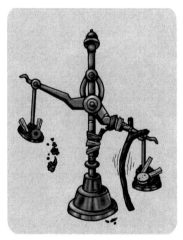

**7 - Loss of Good Nutrients**
A common side effect.

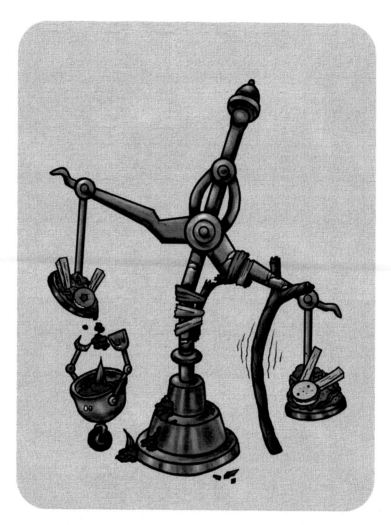

**8 - Off Balance, The American Way of Health**
If you are compliant and listen to your doctor, this is
what your health may eventually look like. The extra
bucket represents the high-tech expensive drugs, that
only work to further maintain the sick, off-balance
state.

## INTERVIEW WITH FORMER PHARMACIST AND ACUPUNCTURIST DR. DENNIS KINNANE

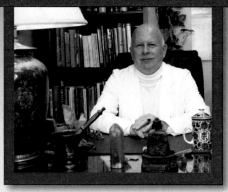

*Dr. Dennis Kinnane, a graduate of Purdue University pharmacy school, worked as a retail pharmacist in chain pharmacies for over 20 years. In 1981, Dr. Kinnane was shocked when what was supposed to be the best of Western medicine failed to save his best friend who passed away from a very common disease at age 35. However, when he learned of a simple herbal remedy that could have saved his friend, he was inspired to change careers and he left the pharmacy profession to pursue Traditional Chinese Medicine (TCM).*

**Dr. Leyla: Why did you go to pharmacy school?**
Dr. Kinnane: My uncle was a pharmacist and I liked pharmacy and being at the drug store. I also liked science and medicine, so I thought it would be a good fit.

**Dr. Leyla: How many years did you spend practicing pharmacy?**
Dr. Kinnane: From 1969 until 1991, I worked at retail drug stores like Sav-on and Thrifty.

**Dr. Leyla: How would you describe the experience?**
Dr. Kinnane: Pharmacy is an old and honorable profession. It has been around for thousands of years. Before modern doctors people would go to the local apothecary or pharmacist who grew and collected herbs and they would create a healing concoction. Nowadays, however, the pharmacists have been steered away from natural therapies and the profession has been hijacked by the pharmaceutical/oil companies. In practice, the days behind the prescription counter were tedious and busy, interrupted with moments of controlled panic from rushed and demanding customers.

**Dr. Leyla: When did you decide to change careers?**
Dr. Kinnane: My best friend died from hepatitis B when he was only 35 years old. I never suspected he would die. He was in one of the most prestigious hospitals in Los Angeles, but after nearly a month he had a massive liver hemorrhage. The doctors didn't do anything for him, only gave him sugar water. After he died I figured that there had to be something that could have helped him. I mean, hepatitis B has been around for years—you mean to tell me that no one has been able to come up with anything?

**Dr. Leyla: So then what happened?**
Dr. Kinnane: Although it was too late for my friend, I read in a herbal book, *The Way of Herbs*[1], that dandelion root, a blood purifier which works in the liver, had been used to treat all kinds of hepatitis including type B for thousands of years. Then one day a customer who had hepatitis B came in the pharmacy asking for some vitamins. I showed them to him, and told him I recently read that dandelion root tea could help. We didn't have any at the drugstore, but later that day he found an herb shop, and bought the tea. I hadn't thought about the interaction again. After a month he came in the pharmacy to thank me. In two weeks of taking the tea his liver tests were normal and his symptoms had subsided. His doctor told him that was impossible.

**Dr. Leyla: Do you mean that an inexpensive, simple, natural product was able to help this customer with a full recovery, while doctors at a prestigious hospital couldn't help your friend?**
Dr. Kinnane: Yes, and the customer paid about $5 for the tea, while my friend's hospital bills were over $150,000 back in 1981. I'm sure that would cost 5 or 10 times more now. That's when I decided to leave pharmacy and enroll in school for Chinese Medicine.

**Dr. Leyla: How did your family and friends react?**
Dr. Kinnane: They thought I was crazy, leaving a good, stable job for Chinese medicine—but I just knew that medicine practiced by billions of people for thousands of years had something to it. My friends and family were discouraging, but once I made up my mind they didn't bother me. I knew it was the path I was supposed to take.

**Dr. Leyla: What did the education consist of?**
Dr. Kinnane: I went to the Samra University of Oriental Medicine for four and a half years to earn first a Master's and then a Doctorate. It was very difficult, as I had to learn an entire new way of thinking, completely different from what's taught in Western science and at pharmacy school. And I had to learn the Chinese culture as well. According to Einstein, matter and energy are interchangeable and transform into one another and that also follows the Chinese theory. However, in Chinese medicine it is the energy or *qi* which is paramount while in Western medicine it is the matter or chemistry which counts most. I had no concept of this when I started.

**Dr. Leyla: What kinds of classes were taught?**
Dr. Kinnane: I had to learn the theory of Chinese internal medicine, acupuncture, how the Chinese view the body as an energetic being, yin and yang as opposite polar forces, herbal medicine, ways to diagnose using tongue and pulse diagnosis, and how to ask the right questions to diagnose.

**Dr. Leyla: As an expert in both the fields, how does Western medicine compare to Chinese Medicine?**
Dr.Kinnane: In pharmacy school, it was explained that we would treat people's symptoms because in many cases there was not yet a cure. It sounds reasonable, but in practice it turns out differently and becomes mostly a long-term suppression of symptoms. Additionally, pharmacy doesn't take into account the element of consciousness; the Chinese call it *qi* or conscious function of an organ, and look at how they interact to keep the body in homeostasis. There is this consciousness that keeps everything functioning properly, and if you take that away you take away the healing power. Chinese medicine views illness as an imbalance or disharmony of organ functions due to *qi* blockage or deficiencies.

Also, one of the problems with Western medicine is that each drug is like a drop of poison. Pharmaceutical drugs are by definition dangerous because they are all toxic. This poison might fix or do good things in some organs, but cause problems, or side effects, in other organs.

Traditional Chinese medicine, on the other hand, is a stand-alone medical model which served the healthcare needs of the Chinese people for over 4000 years. TCM has the capacity to treat any condition we know of. In Western medicine there are always new conditions and diseases, yet in Chinese medicine there are a finite number of organs and therefore a finite number of possible imbalances to treat although the possible symptoms are nearly infinite. This is why we have so much trouble nailing down a disease in Western medicine. We are just focused on symptoms with no understanding of the underlying etiology of these symptoms.

**Dr. Leyla: What kind of conditions do you treat?**
Dr. Kinnane: Although acupuncture is best known for pain relief, I have successfully treated everything from common colds to heart failure over the last 23 years.

**Dr. Leyla: What is the difference between herbs and pharmaceuticals?**
Dr. Kinnane: Pharmaceuticals are single molecules that don't exist in nature. They can't be natural because if they were then you couldn't put a patent on it. Pharmaceutical companies twist it or alter it somehow so they can ensure their profit, but it actually makes it more toxic. Herbs are natural growing products that have medicinal properties. Food is considered a medicine in China.

**Dr. Leyla: What does your initial exam consist of?**
Dr. Kinnane: The patient fills out a thorough questionnaire—to find out which organs are affected. We discuss the questionnaire to get more details of their condition. I then do a tongue and pulse diagnosis. From there I can determine where the imbalance, or stagnation of energy, lies and then I can treat with herbs and acupuncture.

**Dr. Leyla: When do you think TCM is superior to Western medicine?**
Dr. Kinnane: There are lots of conditions that TCM can treat that Western medicine can't seem to touch, or can only create long-term customers.

**Dr. Leyla: In Western medicine, the cause of swelling in the joints, or rheumatoid arthritis, is considered unknown. As you know it's treated with anti-inflammatories, and eventually immune-suppressing drugs leading to side effects and other debilitating problems. How would Chinese medicine treat a patient with rheumatoid arthritis?**

Dr. Kinnane: I go through the symptoms to find out what joints are affected and then we know right away. With Chinese medicine we know that there are three organs of water metabolism, which are spleen, kidney, and lungs. If one or more of these organs are weakened, it can cause the fluid retention and swelling. I find out which organs are not functioning from the exam. Often kidney and spleen are most likely culprits.

**Dr. Leyla: Have you successfully treated rheumatoid arthritis patients?**

Dr. Kinnane: Yes. For example, I had a patient who was on a high dose steroid for 15 years as well as 18 other drugs, and his doctors couldn't get it under control. He had lots of side effects from the steroid, including thinning of his skin, diabetes, osteoporosis, plus two hip replacements and two knee replacements. Additionally his immune system was shot from the steroid, so he was susceptible to infections and other conditions, and therefore had a serious lung infection. I treated him with acupuncture on the meridians of these organs, and an herbal formula. I was able to help him with his rheumatoid arthritis and get him off of many of the medications.

**Dr. Leyla: How is pain treated in Chinese medicine?**

Dr. Kinnane: Pain is *qi* or chi stagnation. If the chi stagnates in the body, we call it pain and if it stagnates too long it can progress to an even worse state called blood stagnation. Pain is treated by removing the cause of the energy blockage with acupuncture and Chinese herbal medicine.

**Dr. Leyla: Does that work with all types of pain, muscle pain, nerve pain, etc.?**

Dr. Kinnane: Yes it works with all types of pain. In TCM there is only chi stagnation or blockage as a cause of pain that needs to be treated.

**Dr. Leyla: What is your best success story?**
Dr. Kinnane: I had a 76 year old heart patient who had arrhythmias, with no two heartbeats the same. He had congestive heart failure and his doctor said that he needed a heart transplant. I found that his spleen and kidneys were weak. When I brought the energy up the heart responded and regained a normal rhythm. This took about a year of work but it lasted for many years afterward. I kept in touch with him. Around his 80th birthday he reroofed his own garage.

**Dr. Leyla: What other services do you provide?**
Dr. Kinnane: I do nutritional consulting based on Chinese dietary energetics; acupressure massage, herbal consultations, and second opinions based on Chinese medicine. I will do evaluations of patient's prescription drugs for interactions and side-effect related illnesses. I teach Yoga techniques for musculoskeletal healing. I also use flower essences to treat certain conditions.

**Dr. Leyla: Are you happy with your career move? Any thoughts of returning to the pharmacy world?**
Dr. Kinnane: I feel that I'm in REAL pharmacy; I feel more of the pharmacist that I expected to become with my herbal pharmacy than I ever did working in a modern drug store dispensing dangerous drugs by the millions every year.

**Dr. Dennis Kinnane**
**4015 Pacific Coast Hwy, Suite 104**
**Torrance, CA  90505**
**(310) 373-9739**

**DrKinnane.com**

DOES YOUR COLON...

LOOK LIKE THIS?

OR LIKE THIS?

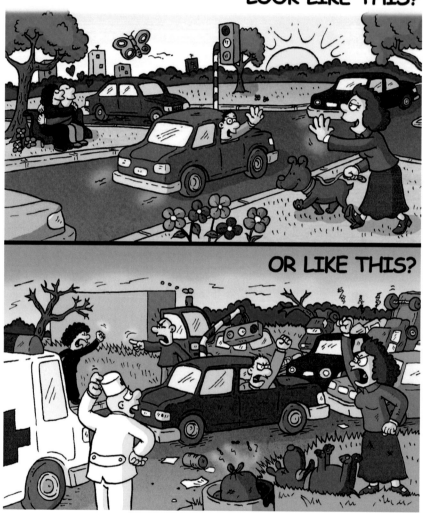

## CHAPTER 5

# CLEANSING AND DETOX

*The system of nature, of which man is a part, tends to be self-balancing, self-adjusting, self-cleansing. Not so with technology.*
*~E.F. Schumacher*

What is cleansing and detoxification? Why would you need to do that?

I did not learn anything about cleansing or detoxification in pharmacy school. The only cleanse that was taught was about the one which is used before a procedure like a colonoscopy. Twelve hours before the examination process, patients must drink four liters of electrolytes. This is available by prescription and it flushes the intestinal system in order to give doctors a clean look inside your colon the next morning.

A few years after my graduation, I was curious about cleansing as it had become trendy, and I was hearing more and more about it. I had a friend who was knowledgeable on the subject, so I asked him about it. He gave me a cleanse kit along with the book *Cleanse and Purify Thyself* [66] by Richard Anderson.

That book was the starting point for my journey of exploring the alternative healthcare options.

**TOXINS**

For thousands of years the world consisted of hunter-gatherers who would scavenge for food such as eggs, nuts, and fruits. Once in a while they would capture an animal and earn their feast. Then, ten thousand years ago, some societies settled down. They set up camp and began planting and harvesting the food they needed.

Just a hundred years ago the world was a much different place:

- Many people grew their own food and purchased other items from local farmers.
- There were no pesticides.
- Cattle ranged on pasture and ate grass before becoming someone's dinner.
- An apple pie was made when apples were in season.
- The air was unpolluted, and people could drink water from streams and wells.
- If someone got sick, there were medical doctors as well as alternative practitioners and healers to choose from.

In today's world:

- Our food is contaminated with pesticides, injected with antibiotics, and genetically modified.
- Cattle stay in substandard conditions and are fed unnatural foods before becoming someone's dinner.
- Our food is pre-packaged, preserved, injected with additives and flavoring, and then frozen before being cooked in a microwave oven.
- One must now go to farmers market, or specialty stores to find organic produce or depend on the small organic section at the local grocery store.
- In many places the air is contaminated with pollutants.
- When someone gets sick, they go to a doctor, who prescribes a medication, which really is another chemical, or another toxin, to treat their condition.
- We can no longer drink from streams or even the faucet as water purifying plants cannot remove all the toxins. Now there are increasing levels of pharmaceuticals found in tap water.[67]

Now our digestive tracts struggle to process everything we ingest, and our lungs struggle to filter the toxins we breathe in.[68]

Is it any wonder that there are an abundance of new health conditions and diseases with causes that are *unknown*?

While our bodies have the ability to detox and remove these toxins (the lymph system, the liver, skin, colon, and blood stream each accomplish this task), they have not evolved as quickly as the amount and variety of chemicals they must now contend with. Quite simply, our bodies are overwhelmed.

Consider the following analogy:

> You are taking a lovely stroll in the park, on a beautiful sunny day. Sitting on a bench, observing your surroundings, your eyes come upon a trashcan, overflowing with garbage. Papers, cans, banana peels, even food containers—it all makes for an unsightly mess.
>
> This eyesore also attracts undesirable scavengers as well as flies due to the growing stench. Without consistent maintenance, this container becomes a bigger and smellier mess, eventually affecting the nearby plants and wildlife negatively.

Our bodies are much the same way.

How does that trash overflow present itself in our bodies? The trash has a nasty stench. Similarly, an unclean interior body can raise a stink, in the form of bad breath and body odor. These are usually caused by the over production of odor-creating bacteria and yeast.

Your body also stores the trashy toxins in your fat and skin cells. This can result in excessive weight gain, and possibly obesity. Your body is always trying to remove toxins through the pores of your skin (an organ of the body), which can cause blemishes, discoloration, dryness, or disease.

The toxins lodged in muscle and organ tissue also wreak havoc on cell health and vitality.[69] The primary function of certain body parts is to process excess solids and fluids in preparation for disposal. Too much of a bad thing can overwhelm the system.

In this case, the liver and kidneys become overworked and their ability to function correctly may be compromised. Over time, damage to the body's filtration and food breakdown process may result in the bowel becoming stressed. If the bowel is unable to do its job properly, the waste is stuck. The results can be constipation, bloating, gas, and pain.

What about those undesirable critters coming around the overflowing trash cans? These compare to unhealthy viruses, bacteria, and even parasites that live and thrive in a toxic body.

## CLEANSING

So how do you treat a body that is a toxic mess?

As previously mentioned, our bodies have several systems, natural body filters, in place to keep toxins out. These include the lymph system, the colon, the lungs, the blood, the liver and the skin.

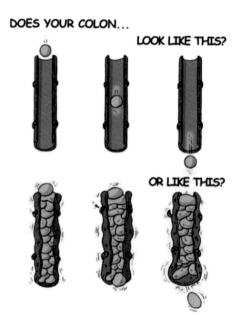

**DOES YOUR COLON...**

**LOOK LIKE THIS?**

**OR LIKE THIS?**

Even though we cleanse ourselves naturally, our body cannot process the sheer volume of toxins that it gets exposed to, voluntarily or not. Because of this, the release of chemicals does not keep pace, resulting in a build up in our tissues and organs.

Here are some different options for cleansing to consider:

- **The Master Cleanse**[70] is pretty simple in form and function. Fresh lemons are mixed with maple syrup and cayenne pepper to drink throughout the day for a few days up to a month. This combination causes the body to neutralize the lemon's acidity by creating an alkaline environment, bringing the body into balance.

- **Raw foods**[71] shift the way your body manages the toxins typically ingested. On a raw food diet, digestion requires minimal acid creation. Other processes break down the foods and the alkaline environment is maintained.

- **Alkaline Water** is a more recent trend. As one might guess, the liquid creates a more alkaline environment in the digestive system, which promotes greater balance to the whole body.

- **Colonic cleansing** is an interesting process, to say the least. According to some naturopaths, 90 percent of diseases are due to improper function of the colon. During a colonic cleanse, a tube is inserted into the rectum, and the patient's intestinal tract is filled with filtered water. Pressure builds as the amount of water increases, which is monitored.

  Then, the flow of water is reversed, the internal pressure eases and the liquid carries excess waste out of the body. The *fill-up-and-release* cycle continues throughout the hour. The provider (and patient) views the outflow through a glass tube, checking for the color, density, texture and abnormalities of the excrement.

  Stories abound of strange and unnatural sightings like pieces of crayon, a marble, and a Barbie doll foot. While undigested food and medication is prevalent, one patient, allergic to penicillin, saw a single dose—a little blue pill—float on by.

- **The Optimal Health Institute**[72] is a facility near San Diego, CA. Their program requires a one-week minimum stay, where the focus is to cleanse and purify the body, mind and spirit. Each day consists of a raw food diet, a detoxifying exercise class, meditation, and daily classes that educate about and support the program. Enemas are also part of the regimen and colonics are available as an option.

The Institute has been in existence for thirty years. People go there with a variety of conditions, including cancer. Health conditions are referred to as "health opportunities," as they give people the *opportunity* to step out of their daily routine and seek greater health and balance than they would otherwise—on a physical, emotional, and spiritual level.

- **Juice fasts**[73] are done by drinking only fresh juice for 24 to 72 hours, or even longer. They give the digestive system a rest and help detoxify on a regular basis.

- **Natural products** like organic produce, soaps, and deodorants are good options so the body doesn't get exposed to additional toxins.

There are many ways to cleanse. In the past, the air we breathed and the food we ate were cleaner and more pure. Our bodies had enough resources to fend off the invaders and could use their own natural processes to cleanse. Now our bodies are overwhelmed with pollutants and toxins, and therefore may need some help in removing them.

## ACID-BASE BALANCE

We often hear about the acid-base balance in the body. There is an optimal acidity level for the different parts of the body, and these are directly affected by what we eat.

To follow the digestion of food, when food is swallowed it travels down the esophagus and then to the stomach, which is the most acidic part of the body. The extra acid serves to break down the food to help the digestion process. After passing through the stomach the food then goes to the intestines, which is much more alkaline and prepares the food further for absorption.

Whole and raw foods are easier for our bodies to breakdown, and therefore produce less acid than meat or processed foods. Meat and processed foods require the stomach to create more acid to help break down and digest the food. However, when a person eats processed food or meat daily for months or years, the body can get overwhelmed with this increased amount of acid, which over time will affect the surrounding tissues and organs. Eventually the intestines can no longer maintain an alkaline environment, and this can lead to vulnerability to a variety of conditions and diseases.

The common denominator in most of the previously mentioned cleanses is they work to remove toxins and get the body into a less acidic and more alkaline state. The foods we eat can work to get us in a healthier, less toxic state. According to naturopaths, more than 95 percent of all diseases are caused by what we eat.[74] By choosing foods that don't cause the stomach to create an abundance of acid, we can stay in a healthier, more alkaline, and disease-free state.

The following chart provides an overview of which foods create an acidic environment and which create a more alkaline environment.

| FOOD CATEGORY | High Alkaline | Alkaline | Low Alkaline | Low Acid | Acid | High Acid |
|---|---|---|---|---|---|---|
| BEANS, VEGETABLES, LEGUMES | Vegetable Juices, Parsley, Raw Spinach, Broccoli, Celery, Barley Grass, Garlic | Carrots, Green Beans, Lima Beans, Beets, Lettuce, Zucchini, Carob | Squash, Asparagus, Fresh Corn, Onions, Peas, Cauliflower, Potato, Olives, Tofu | Sweet Potato, Cooked Spinach, Kidney Beans | Pinto Beans, Navy Beans | Pickled Vegetables |
| FRUIT | Dried Figs, Raisins | Dates, Black-currents, Grapes, Papaya, Kiwi, Berries, Apples, Pears | Coconut, Tomatoes, Oranges, Cherries, Pineapple, Avocados, Grapefruit, Strawberries, Watermelon, Lemons, Limes | Bluberries, Cranberries, Bananas, Plums, Processed Fruit Juices | Canned Fruit | |
| GRAINS, CEREALS | | | Amaranth, Lentils, Wild Rice, Quinoa, Millet | Rye Bread, Whole Grain Bread, Oats, Brown Rice | White Rice, White Bread, Pastries, Biscuits, Pasta | |
| MEAT | | | | Liver, Oysters, Organ Meat | Fish, Turkey, Chicken, Lamb | Beef, Pork, Veal, Shellfish, Canned Tuna & Sardines |
| EGGS & DAIRY | | Breast Milk | Soy Cheese, Soy Milk, Whey, Goat Cheese, Buttermilk | Whole Milk, Butter, Yogurt, Cottage Cheese, Cream, Ice Cream | Eggs, Camembert, Hand Cheese | Parmesan, Processed Cheese |
| NUTS & SEEDS | | Hazelnuts, Almonds | Chestnuts, Brazils, Coconut | Pumpkin, Sesame, Sunflower Seeds | Pecans, Cashews, Pistachios | Peanuts, Walnuts |
| OILS | | | Flax-Seed Oil, Olive Oil, Canola Oil | Corn Oil, Sunflower Oil, Margarine, Lard | | |
| BEVERAGES | Herb Teas, Lemon Water | Green Tea | Ginger Tea | Cocoa | Wine, Soda/Pop | Tea (black), Coffee, Beer, Liquor |
| SWEETENERS, CONDIMENTS | Stevia | Maple Syrup, Rice Syrup | Raw Honey, Raw Sugar | White Sugar, Processed Honey | Milk Chocolate, Brown Sugar, Molasses, Ketchup, Mayonnaise | Artificial Sweeteners |

## ACID-BASE CHEMISTRY

To go a step further, we can look at the chemistry behind the acid-base balance. This section provides a simple, clear understanding of what acid and base balance is at a chemical level, and its importance to a healthy human body.

1. pH stands for potential for hydrogen, which is a measure of the acid or alkaline levels of a solution. Different parts of the body have different pH levels. The stomach is the most acidic place in the body.

2. The chemical nature of water is $H_2O$. Each water molecule consists of one-part oxygen and two-parts hydrogen. The connections look like this:

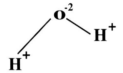

- Hydrogen particles have a +1 charge

- Oxygen particles have a -2 charge
  - H (+1) + H (+1) = +2 (two hydrogens)
    - O (-2) = _-2 (plus one oxygen)
      0

- Therefore, two particles of hydrogen combined with one particle of oxygen creates a neutral charge

The water molecule's equation is net zero, giving us a neutral and stable compound.

3. Acidic, by definition, is an excess of hydrogen particles (H+) ready to react. When something is acidic it means that

77

there is an excess of hydrogen *in the mix.* Once again, the human body is always trying to maintain balance.

| ACIDIC | MORE ACIDIC |
|--------|-------------|
| $H^{+1}$ $H^{+1}$ $H^{+1}$ $H^{+1}$ $H^{+1}$ $H^{+1}$ | $H^{+1}$ $H^{+1}$$H^{+1}$ $H^{+1}$ $H^{+1}$ $H^{+1}$ $H^{+1}$ $H^{+1}$ $H^{+1}$ $H^{+1}$ $H^{+1}$ $H^{+1}$ $H^{+1}$ $H^{+1}$ $H^{+1}$ $H^{+1}$ $H^{+1}$ $H^{+1}$ $H^{+1}$ $H^{+1}$ $H^{+1}$ $H^{+1}$ |

$$(OH-) + (H+) = 0$$

4.  Did you ever wonder what happens when alcohol is consumed? The chemical nature of alcohol (OH-) is 1-part oxygen (-2 charge) and 1-part hydrogen (+1 charge). Therefore, alcohol (OH-) carries a negative one (-1) charge.

All alcohol products have a (-1) charge. So when we consume alcohol, the body's natural response is to neutralize the chemical imbalance introduced into the system. It will attempt to do so by producing more hydrogen particles:

$$OH^{-1} \ + \ H^{+1} \longrightarrow H_2O$$

| DRINK ALCOHOL | BODY RESPONDS BY PRODUCING ACID | REACT TO CREATE WATER |
|---------------|---------------------------------|-----------------------|

So, when a person drinks alcohol, the body responds by creating more acid (H+) in the stomach. It is not uncommon for some people to experience reflux, or burning in the esophagus, when drinking. This is the body's overreaction of producing hydrogen particles in attempt to neutralize the alcohol.

The American diet is overwhelmingly sourced from processed foods—cooked, pre-prepared, packaged, salted, sweetened—and this automatically puts our stomachs to work.

Many foods, especially those industrially-produced, focus on *texture and flavor* rather than ease of digestion. The more acid that is necessary to break down the foods we eat, the greater the acidic environment in the stomach from which our bloodstream distributes nourishment, and this eventually leads to more acidity of the entire body.

The body risks developing chronic pH imbalance which, over decades, can affect its ability to properly function. According to naturopathic medicine, the foods we eat can create an acidic environment, and it is this acidic state that is the precursor of many diseases suffered today. The processed food and foods with artificial ingredients cause the stomach to make too much acid, which can increase the risk of many diseases.

Given this theory, most diseases can be cured by dramatically changing how we eat: by switching from processed foods and meats, to those natural foods of a plant-based diet that do not create excess acid.

Holistic practitioners and naturopaths understand that raw food does not require excessive levels of stomach acid in order to be digested. The opportunity to maintain a healthy pH balance is available to all. However, the motive for most food production is taste and profit, rather than health.

Interesting tidbit: we all recognize that lemons are high in acid content, as are most citrus foods. Put a lemon in your mouth for 10 seconds, and then measure inside your mouth for pH level, or acidity level. Most people would expect to find that the mouth is more acidic after the lemons. The opposite is actually true. The body quickly responds, in its attempt to neutralize the acid, and thus the pH of your mouth would be more alkaline.

## *IN CONCLUSION:*

Americans consume massive quantities of food that are unnatural for our bodies to digest. Although the existence of acid in the  stomach is normal, the body responds to processed food and foods with artificial ingredients by creating an excess of acid in the stomach and eventually the entire body. This translates to increased risk of poor health and chronic disease.

## POINTS TO REMEMBER:

- Because of the food we eat and the toxic world we live in, it is advisable to cleanse our bodies internally.

- Doctors and pharmacists are not trained on cleansing and detoxification.

- Most detoxification diets and cleanses work by changing your body to a less acidic and more alkaline state.

- Many health conditions can be remedied by changing the foods that we eat.

## INTERVIEW WITH HOLISTIC HEALTH PRACTITIONER STORM COLE

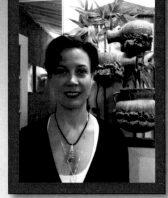

*Storm Cole is a former dance instructor with a diverse background in sports as well as in the arts. At age 22 years she was diagnosed with fibromyalgia and chronic fatigue, and also suffered heavy metal poisonings. Her family doctor offered no solutions or treatment; he only mocked her complaint.*

*Storm found her healing through holistic and natural approaches. Now she dedicates her life to well-being as a holistic health practitioner, helping others reestablish their health and regain balance through nutritional counseling, blood-cell analysis, full-body scanning, and other methods.*

**Dr. Leyla: What was your life like before your health conditions?**
Storm: I was a dancer and a student at CSU Long Beach. I also taught modern dance, ballet, and hip hop.

**Dr. Leyla: What kind of health conditions did you have?**
Storm: I had multiple herniated discs that would randomly deteriorate due to poor protein digestion, my spine was weak (probably from emotional stress), and I had a flesh eating virus that went into my shoulder. I was disabled for a year; I wasn't able to teach. Also, my valves would blow in the ileum of my stomach, and I would have problems with my digestion. To make things even worse, waste matter from my colon would get into my blood. My eyes would turn black. My thyroid would be off, so I was often freezing cold. The toxins in my blood, or toxemia, caused my blood to be sticky, taxing my heart.

**Dr. Leyla: What do you believe was the underlying cause of your health conditions?**
Storm: From a medical standpoint, I had chronic fatigue, fibromyalgia, and strep infections. From a holistic standpoint, I was having too much

emotional stress, mostly from not having boundaries and doing too much for people. I was not setting limits and I was being taken advantage of. I had a type 1 personality: *yes, I can do it all, and I might even do it for free.*

**Dr. Leyla: Regarding the chronic fatigue, what types of symptoms did you experience?**
Storm: I could sleep for 12 hours, then wake up and be completely exhausted. I had brain fog. I couldn't remember people's names, or what I've done. I was singing then, but I never knew what my voice would sound like. I had pain, pain, pain. All over pain, everything hurt. I could feel the cells and all my cells were screaming.

**Dr. Leyla: What other complications did you have?**
Storm: Besides the chronic fatigue, I had flesh eating bacteria in my shoulder and I couldn't use it for a year. I also had herniated discs. I couldn't break down protein so the food became bricks going through my body. There was nothing holding me together. And I was in a bad mood, and mean. Nobody likes you when you have a bad, miserable attitude. I was craving bad food which continued the downward spiral into a snowball. Also, my immune system was dysfunctional, as my whole system was distorted. I was vulnerable to other conditions and the doctors had no cure.

**Dr. Leyla: How long were you like that?**
Storm: For six years my condition was getting progressively worse.

**Dr. Leyla: Did a doctor diagnose you?**
Storm: Initially I did my own research on the internet and came to the conclusion that I had chronic fatigue. I went to my doctor, who was a friend of my family for years. He actually laughed at me; he said that he had chronic fatigue too, isn't it funny? He thought it was in my head.

**Dr. Leyla: How did you react to that?**
Storm: I was pissed, hurt, and disgusted really. I had known him for years and he knew that I wasn't one to go to a doctor for minor symptoms

or problems. I was frustrated because I knew that I was feeling horrible and something was very wrong, but there was no medical test to confirm it.

**Dr. Leyla: So what did you do after that?**
Storm: I was analyzed by a naturopath who agreed it was chronic fatigue. I was so relieved because she was empathetic. She understood the pain and that there was something wrong. She started with contact reflex analysis, which is muscle testing on different points on the body to determine if the condition was systemic.

**Dr. Leyla: How would you describe the healing?**
Storm: I would make improvements and take three steps up, then plateau. Then three steps up and then plateau. At some point you forget how bad you ever felt.

**Dr. Leyla: How did you treat the chronic fatigue?**
Storm: It took two to three years to get totally cleaned up. During that time I did emotional clearing, used essential oils, and used Emotional Freedom Technique (EFT). Much of my physical condition was caused by emotional distress. Because I wasn't setting boundaries, I would let myself get taken advantage of financially, and I wouldn't stand up for myself. I wondered what was wrong with me.

I used the power of forgiveness, of myself and of others, which is one of the most divine things you can do. It's a matter of letting go, and according to holistic therapies, it is the cause of all conditions. It brings you back to God, otherwise it's about ego and you have to get past that. The naturopathic practitioner used contact reflex analysis, and went over my body to check for what was wrong. I also took Standard Process Products, which are whole foods in pill form, to give your body the nutrients that it's lacking.

**Dr. Leyla: Regarding the herniated discs, what kind of symptoms did you experience?**
Storm: I had severe pain in the back, couldn't walk, and couldn't dance.

**Dr. Leyla: Medical doctors would treat a herniated disc with pain killers, physical therapy, or surgery. What kind of treatment did your doctor offer?**
Storm: I never went back to the doctor after that first diagnosis because it was clear I wasn't going to get anything I needed from him.

**Dr. Leyla: How did you treat your herniated discs?**
Storm: The naturopath gave me enzymes because the proteins weren't being broken down, so my body couldn't regenerate itself. I also had to clean out my digestive system with enzymes. I had to let go of some favorite foods, including wheat, cheese, sugars, and dairy, in order to reboot and tone up my body. I took high protein capsules to help the tissues regenerate themselves.

**Dr. Leyla: And then after you recovered from those issues, you had another health challenge. What happened?**
Storm: I got chemical poisoning from heavy metals and herbicides and pesticides. My neighbor had tall bushes to keep us separated. He sprayed pesticides all over. My cat died because of it.

**Dr. Leyla: What kind of symptoms did you experience?**
Storm: It was hard for me to breathe. I had no stamina and I had chemical burns on my skin. My entire body was bloated, I had liver dysfunction, joint pain, nerve pain, and digestion was poor to struggling. I gained weight because my body was unable to breakdown food, and I had a huge lump in my stomach. It was like Chernobyl happened inside my body.

**Dr. Leyla: How did you deal with this?**
Storm: At this point I was much more aware of what I needed to do to heal. I used Standard Process products to cleanse.

**Dr. Leyla: At what point did you decide to become a holistic practitioner?**
Storm: I decided after I finished massage school. With massage I was helping people feel better, but I wasn't getting them better. I knew I could

do so much more, especially since I had been through so much with my own health.

**Dr. Leyla: What type of conditions do you treat?**
Storm: I treat people with chronic fatigue, Lyme disease, hiatal hernia, and autoimmune disorders.

**Dr. Leyla: How do you evaluate the patients?**
Storm: I do a blood analysis. With the blood analysis, we work with both live and dried blood. Live-blood nutritional analysis looks at what is happening in your body today. Of course one could see all sorts of things that a doctor can see, but we are only allowed to note the nutritional variables. This is done with one drop of blood that is then put on a screen and observed with a microscope. There's a large monitor so the client can see the blood cells as well. Smokers are the most interested in their blood because the cell damage is so rampant that it really inspires them to make changes. Some examples of things I would be allowed to note in the blood are cholesterol, inability to digest fat, free-radical damage, iron deficiency, hormonal imbalance, etc. Dried blood shows your history. If you've had head or spine trauma in the past it will show here. If your lymphatics are backed up, or you've had or are moving towards cancer, this is where you will see it. I don't think we can say that, but we would refer you to a doctor. Heavy metals, environmental issues, and vitamin and mineral deficiency will also show here. Dried blood analysis is done with one finger prick, but you need seven drops of blood from the one prick.

**Dr. Leyla: What is the NES machine?**
Storm: The Nutri-Energetics System (NES) machine reads your human body field through the hand scanner and compares it to average healthy bodies in your age range. It detects blocks, and damage in the acupuncture meridians, chakras, auric fields, tissues, emotions, and the musculoskeletal system. It also notes your susceptibility to environmental toxins, and your ability to utilize nutrients. The NES family is always working on improving their equipment. Now the NES system also shows where and how to recover the fields of old traumas that

may show up and cause problems or haunt you—today or possibly in the future.

**Dr. Leyla: Once you find the problem, or imbalance, how can you treat the patients?**
Storm: First treat them with compassion. Second, ask how their body heals best. Let them know that their feedback is vital, then decide if you want to work nutritional to emotional, electrical to spiritual, energetic to sleep rhythms. Everyone is going to be so different; there is no set protocol.

**Dr. Leyla: What if you didn't find holistic practitioners and you only relied upon medical doctors for your health conditions. How do you think your life would be today?**
Storm: I would be on disability or dead.

**Dr. Leyla: How is your life today?**
Storm: My life today is great. I'm human; I still get things like the cold or flu, but nothing like before. My awareness of everything, from a plant, to myself, is much greater and I'm very thankful for that.

**Dr. Leyla: What is it that people need to know that they don't learn from their doctor?**
Storm: I think it is important to know that there is always hope. And that you will not find a one-week cure. Don't give up, and don't try something and then go to the next and the next. It takes the body four months to turn over every cell inside it, so trying something for one or two weeks isn't realistic.

**Storm Cole, BA, HHP**
**5018 Katella Ave., Los Alamitos, CA  90720**
**storm@stormcolehhp.com**
**(562) 972-1235**

**StormColeHHP.com**

# I LOST 140 POUNDS IN TWO WEEKS! THANKS NOFATIN!

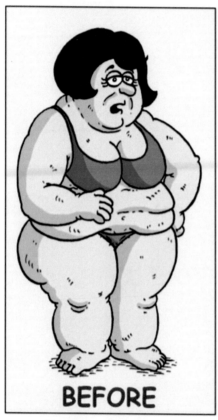

BEFORE

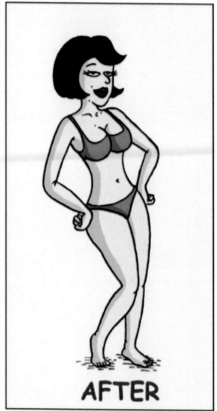

AFTER

RESULTS NOT TYPICAL.
RESULTS MAY BE REVERSIBLE.
YOU MAY ACTUALLY BECOME FATTER THAN WHEN YOU STARTED.
OTHER SIDE EFFECTS INCLUDE: HEADACHE, NAUSEA, AGITATION, DIARRHEA,
UNCONTROLLABLE BOWEL ACTIVITY, ANAL LEAKAGE, MEMORY LOSS, HEART FAILURE,
SEIZURES, DEPRESSION, DECREASED LIBIDO, BAD BREATH, AND EARLY DEATH.
PLEASE DISCUSS WITH YOUR DOCTOR IF NOFATIN IS RIGHT FOR YOU.

## CHAPTER 6

# WEIGHT LOSS

*Let Food Be Thy Medicine and Medicine Be They Food.*
*~Hippocrates*

When I was a kid, there weren't many overweight people. Everyone in school was thin except for the random kid that stuck out like a sore thumb. Things have changed since then:

- The food has changed.
- Our activities have changed.
- Even the way we eat has changed, as sit down dinners are often the exception rather than the rule.

We've all seen the statistics:

- Obesity is a growing problem with more people becoming obese all the time.
- We see the commercials showing pictures of fat bellies while hiding the faces to maintain anonymity.
- The majority of us know that obesity is associated with diabetes, heart problems, and early death.

So what new information can I possibly share?

## DEFINITION

Obesity is defined as abnormal or excessive fat accumulation that presents a risk to health. The body mass index (BMI) is a formula created to classify and categorize one's level of obesity. BMI is a person's weight (in kilograms) divided by the square of his or her height (in meters). A person with a BMI of 25 to 30 is considered overweight, and if the BMI is over 30 the person is considered obese.[75]

## STATISTICS

How many people are overweight? According to the World Health Organization (WHO):[76]

- Worldwide obesity has more than doubled since 1980.
- In 2008, 1.4 billion adults, 20 years of age and older, were overweight. Of these, over 200 million men and nearly 300 million women were obese.
- Sixty-five percent of the world's population lives in countries where being overweight or obese kills more people than being underweight.
- Nearly 40 million children under the age of five were overweight in 2010.

## INDUSTRY

With over two-thirds of the population classified as obese, the dieting industry has earned huge profits becoming an annual $55 billion industry, selling diets, videos, books, and other weight loss products.[77]

## HEALTH RISKS

Obesity is a major risk factor for a variety of chronic diseases including diabetes, heart disease, and cancer. Arthritis, high blood pressure and high cholesterol are also more prevalent. The excess weight and physical appearance can also have negative effects on emotional health, which can lead to depression and anxiety.[78]

**90**

## *GLOBESITY*

Since it has become such a growing problem, literally, the WHO now refers to the global epidemic of overweight and obese humans as *globesity*.[79]

The number of obese people continues to increase, despite the new diets and miracle drugs that are consistently flowing to market.

But the fact is, the cycle of putting your body into a mode of starvation, or eating bland foods while your body is craving everything else, is simply not the healthy approach to well-being that the human body needs. In fact, it fits the standard medical and pharmaceutical model as a ***temporary solution with negative, long-term side effects,*** which include stronger cravings and gaining more weight than before the diet.

Additionally, the pharmaceutical industry has profited from its own money-making drugs. The drugs companies participate by developing miracle pills, both prescription and over-the-counter, to promote the so-called *cure.*

There are many diet plans, in the form of pill regimens, which gained significant traction in America, yet failed as solutions to obesity. Difficulties arose only after the fact, whether in the form of inability to maintain healthy weight levels, or damage to the human body. Both scenarios often resulted in pounds regained and the emotional damage after, once again, failing a diet.

## DRUGS FOR OBESITY

### Phen-Fen

Many may remember the phen-fen fad in the 1990s.[80] There was a significant advertising buzz when it was promoted as the perfect combination of two drugs, phentermine and fenfluramine. Each worked with a different mechanism of action to reduce weight, and the side effects of each drug were opposite of each other, and thus would cancel each other out.

Well, it was *supposed* to be perfect.

> **Phentermine** is basically a prescription form of speed. It is a stimulant that causes nervousness, irritability, insomnia, agitation, dizziness, dry mouth, constipation, elevated blood pressure, and rapid or irregular heartbeats.

> **Fenfluramine** stimulates the release of extra serotonin in the body, which gives the feeling of being full and satisfied. Side effects include drowsiness, sedation, diarrhea, and depression.

The combination of the two drugs was expected to be a huge success. In reality, the effects of drugs on the body are often not understood until long after market acceptance. With phen-fen, over six million people had taken the drug combination before it was found to cause valvular heart disease and pulmonary hypertension, causing heart problems and death in some patients.[81]

In normal functioning, the heart valve closes, pressure increases, and then the next valve opens so blood can be shot into the bloodstream with enough force to meet the body's demands for oxygen. This is important since oxygen is a necessary ingredient for cell survival and must be distributed throughout the entire body.

In valvular heart disease, the valves do not close properly and the required pressure is not reached, thus the blood cannot be pumped as forcefully through the body as necessary. The FDA received over 100 reports of valvular heart disease in phen-fen patients. On July 8th, 1997, the manufacturer voluntarily pulled it off the market. Thirty percent of the patients who were evaluated presented with abnormal valve function.[82] There have been more than 50,000 product responsibility lawsuits submitted by victims of phen-fen.[83]

This was yet another case where the desired effects are immediate, but the side effects and problems develop over the years. All drugs have side effects, and many are discovered only after a large number of patients have taken the drug.

## Thyroid Hormones

The thyroid gland is largely responsible for metabolism. When a patient's thyroid gland is not producing enough thyroid hormone, then often the doctor will prescribe a thyroid replacement tablet to compensate. Using thyroid tablet for weight loss also seemed like another grand idea, as thyroid hormones are natural hormones in the body. Initially, they worked well until it was recognized that patients were losing a lot of calcium and nitrogen. The weight loss experienced was actually coming from lean body tissue rather than fat. Additionally, as the patient was ingesting an outside source of thyroid hormone, the gland itself responded by reducing the amount of hormone it naturally produced. In its effort to maintain balance, the thyroid gland produced less, then atrophied, or weakened, and after time could completely stop working. There were additional side effects, including elevated heart beat, arrhythmias, even sudden death. To add insult to thyroid injury, when the drug is discontinued the weight is quickly regained.[84]

## Meridia

Meridia works by inhibiting the uptake of serotonin and norepinephrine, thus the patient feels satisfied and appetite is decreased. Side effects include insomnia, constipation, dry mouth, increased blood pressure, and seizures. Although Meridia never created a big hype as some other weight loss drugs and products, it was on the market for a while until a study suggested that it may cause more cardiovascular side effects such as heart attack or stroke. In October, 2010 the manufacturer pulled it off the market.[85]

## Alli

Alli is one of more recent drugs to arrive on the market, and it does not require a prescription. The huge advertising push for the drug generated lots of hype. I remember the pharmacies couldn't keep it on the shelves at first. The premise is that by taking this pill, the user can prevent fat from being absorbed in the body during the digestive process. Since the drug works in the stomach, and does not get absorbed in the bloodstream, then the manufacturer can advertise that there are minimal *systemic* side effects. However, there are some troublesome gastrointestinal side effects. These side effects include:

- The inability to absorb fat. Therefore, fat soluble vitamins will not be absorbed. These include vitamins A, D, E, and K as well as beta-carotene.
- Gas with oily spotting (or anal leakage).
- Loose stools.
- More frequent stools; possibly hard to control.

According to the manufacturer:

*"This excess fat that passes out of your body is not harmful. In fact, you may recognize it as something that looks like the oil on top of a pizza. Eating a low-fat diet lowers the chance of these bowel changes. Limit fat intake in your meals to an average of 15 grams."*[86]

Put simply, Alli works by blocking fat absorption. If you eat fatty food, the fat will not be absorbed in the stomach. So where does it go? It will have to exit the body somehow, and this is when it can get messy.

Additionally, although Alli claimed to offer no "systemic side effects," in August 2009 the FDA put out a warning after reports of severe liver injury.[87]

In conclusion, if you are overweight and uncomfortable, Alli might be the answer for you. But if being overweight isn't enough of a drag, now you may have to suffer through gaseous episodes that involve "oily spotting." Additionally, this miracle weight loss pill isn't enough by itself; it must be administered with a diet plan in order to achieve maximum benefit. So remember to exercise and eat right.

## Hoodia

Hoodia has been on the scene for miracle weight loss for quite some time with a bonus of being "all natural." The story of its origin was that it was used in the Kalahari Desert as a natural appetite suppressant. Indigenous peoples were able to survive long treks in the parched-climate expanse while ingesting this wondrous ingredient.

This plant-based extract has appetite suppression qualities that minimize feeling hungry. Similar to other drugs and products, when combined with *healthy food choices*, and *consistent* exercise, Hoodia can help a person lose weight.

Although most sources claim that there are no extreme side effects, some sites are mentioning potential problems with the liver. The fact is that until a greater number of people try it, the effectiveness and side effects may not be known for many years.[88]

## HUMAN CHORIONIC GONADOTROPIN (hCG)

Human Chorionic gonadotropin (hCG) is a pregnancy hormone that must be injected, and the latest diet trend to hit the market. hCG works by *mobilizing fat stores* and using the fat for energy. A strict 500 calorie diet is also necessary. Side effects include those symptoms associated with being pregnant, such as swelling, breast tenderness and water retention. There are no serious side effects reported. However, weight loss can very likely be from the 500 calorie diet rather than hCG. With all drugs, more side effects may be discovered as time passes and more patients take the drug.[89]

## LAP-BAND AND STOMACH SURGERY

LAP-BAND® and stomach surgery are the latest and greatest trends for weight loss, and are now advertised on billboards, television commercials, and magazines. They work by reducing the amount of food that the stomach can hold, therefore causing the patients to eat less and lose weight. As an added bonus, this procedure is covered by many insurance plans.

Although patients are said to lose between 48 to 98 pounds in first year, as with any surgery there are potential complications. Some people experience nutritional deficiencies, while others can regain all their weight back. There are now limitations on the amount and types of foods that can be eaten. An expensive surgery that will cut into your body and lead to other potential problems should never be the first choice to lose weight.[90]

## WEIGHT LOSS PRODUCTS, PLANS, AND PROGRAMS

Visit any food store, vitamin shop, or simply turn on the TV and you will see displays and advertisements promoting weight loss. Previously these efforts were primarily geared towards women, but it's now sexy and masculine for men to join a whole host of diet plans as well—just bring your checkbook.

Advertisers would like you to believe that these programs are safe and effective, and that it would be silly to assume the providers are motivated solely by your wallet. This is a profit-seeking endeavor. As long as individuals desire the quick fix—only to fall off the required regimen later on, and probably gain more weight—the business of weight loss will thrive.

So, here's something to consider: why not gain a piece of this multi-billion dollar action? I have cracked the code in creating a diet or weight loss program that can attract the right buzz, sell like hotcakes and earn millions!

**The Four Easy Steps to Create the Weight Loss Program that will earn MILLIONS!**

1. **Promote Exercise.** Simply suggest a 20-minute daily walk, or better yet create a DVD. Possibly include a detailed workout regimen. Bottom line, mention exercise.

2. **Provide a Sample Diet.** Display your ideal day with a detailed breakdown of what's to eat. Multiple sample eating plans, at least five, is optimal. It should look and sound delicious and fattening. For gangbuster profits, include recipes (for sale) of easy-to-prepare food items.

3. **Create a Product or Routine.** This is where you can promote a pill, a program, or an exercise plan. The key here is to develop the idea/vision so it *sounds* unique. It's imperative to insert the all-important disclaimer: "Must follow the prescribed diet and exercise regimen."

4. **Create the Hype.** Photographs of actual clients, before and after their experience, always work. Make sure both photos are eye catching, one in terms of gross beginnings; the other showing the miracle result. With a little extra investment of time and money, infomercials have a great track record of generating sales. Wave in a celebrity to gain even more attention, and you possibly have an ideal scenario for success. Don't forget to add the disclaimer "Results Not Typical."

Almost all diet and weight loss plans on the market have these standard ingredients to success. The fact is that most, if not all, diets work as long as the person sticks to the prescribed and/or unnatural regimen. Just as pills provide temporary solutions and significant profits for manufacturers, most diet plans are created to make a profit by offering the buyer a quick solution to their problem.

The reality of diet, wellness, weight gain or loss, and fitness has *everything* to do with thoughts, emotions, and attitude. The human condition is well understood by marketers: the more often we're told that we can't have something, the more we crave it. Dieting involves lack, and to survive without something, one must *be strong, stick to the plan, and don't give up!* Military cadets in boot camp are trained to stay energized physically and emotionally to deal with pressure in order to survive at their highest potential. Diets have a similar approach. Most humans cannot maintain this level of intensity forever. It's simply not natural or sustainable. Many feel so deprived that when they do cheat it has snowball effect and becomes a purge, gaining even more weight than before they started the diet. This, unfortunately, feeds right into the business model for the producers of these pills and programs.

## PROBLEMS WITH PAST WEIGHT LOSS TREATMENTS

- After trying diet after diet, or yo-yo dieting, people are getting fatter in the long run. The diets work for a while, but once off the diet then often people gain all their weight back plus more. This is due to the starvation mode. Our bodies have a set point, which is a *natural* weight that the body strives to maintain. Starvation diets with minimal calories push the natural set point to a higher weight, which serves to protect ourselves from actual starvation. This stems from the days of hunter and gatherer, when people would go for a long time without food.[91]

- Diets rely on high motivation and resistance of cravings. It's not natural to fight urges all the time and be in a constant state of struggle. When one finally gives in to the cravings, often the entire house of cards falls as well.

- Most don't deal with underlying emotions that contribute to being overweight.

- Often the drugs are toxic and cause side effects and complications, as we've seen with phen-fen, Meridia, and thyroid tablets.

## WHAT REALLY WORKS?

Now that we've gone over all the problems and limitations of common diet pills and programs, how should one really lose weight?

**Deal with Emotions.** Often there is an emotional cause behind overeating. Learning how to deal with these emotions is a step in the right direction.

**Overeater's Anonymous.** The sister organization of Alcoholics Anonymous, this programs helps people lose weight by following their 12-step guidelines, including admitting powerlessness, turning their lives over to god, as well as dealing with emotions.

It includes "...making a list of all persons we had harmed" and making "direct amends to such people wherever possible, except when to do so would injure them or others."[92]

**Aim for a Natural Release of the Weight.**  Set an intention to discover and deal with the underlying cause of the excess pounds, and the weight will be naturally released.

**Taste Your Food.**  People often eat unconsciously—they're rushed or possibly distracted, watching television, or working on the computer while downing a bag of chips.  Many people will dream about, or crave a certain food.  Yet when they finally eat it they feel guilty and stuff it down their throat, barely tasting it. Slowing down and consciously eating food to enjoy the taste and pleasure of it is another important step to losing weight naturally.

Check out Alfonso de Rose's ThinnerJourney™ at AlfonsodeRose. com, which includes seminars in which people learn how to be open, to enjoy the pleasure of their food, and learn how to be alive, among other things to create a natural release of weight.[93]

**Good Thoughts While Eating.**  The energy that you have while you are eating is very important.  Are you relaxed?  Are you feeling guilty because of what you are eating?  What are your thoughts? Is the food going exactly where it needs to go to nourish the body? Or are you eating as quickly as possible?

**Cleansing.**  Getting rid of toxins and eating a more natural, plant-based diet.  The processed, factory-made foods we eat can be stored in the fat cells and make it more difficult to lose weight.

**Nutrition.**  Most people eat lots of foods that have no nutritional value—or empty calories.  Often we are still hungry because we are lacking the nutrition that our body craves.  Eating superfoods, or foods packed with nutrition that your body needs, will help reduce cravings and help in overall health and wellbeing.

**Loving Yourself.**  Loving yourself as you are, inside and out, and completely, is an important step in allowing the weight to fall off naturally.

## SUMMARY

Dieting, like the other parts of our healthcare system, has followed the lines of creating quick fixes and temporary solutions that appeal to the masses, but cause more problems down the line.

Diet fads have made billions for the industry as the population has grown in weight and obesity at epidemic proportions.

In the past, healthy and lean folks maintained their status via hyped-up motivations towards exercise, food measurements, and calorie intake. The mantra was simple: GO, GO, GO! YOU CAN DO IT. The diet was as successful as your will power. Yet dieters end up with bad feelings after trying diet after diet, and failing.

However, the future success of becoming healthy and lean will be based on being comfortable in our bodies, having internal gratitude for the bounty which surrounds us, being naturally lean because we know and appreciate limits, eating foods rich in nutrition, letting go of past guilt, and dealing with emotions. Out with the struggle, and in with inner peace.

## POINTS TO REMEMBER:

- Obesity is a huge and growing problem.

- Most people fail standard diets and regain weight.

- Like many drugs, diets often create profit and provide a very limited and temporary solution, and rarely address the underlying or emotional cause.

- To successfully maintain a healthy weight, issues beyond diet and exercise must be addressed, including emotions, thoughts, cleansing, and nutrition.

## INTERVIEW WITH EMOTIONAL EATING SPECIALIST
## RAQUEL REYNA

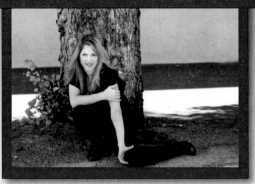

*Raquel competed in gymnastics at the young age of eight. Her weight was constantly monitored to the point that she was often told she was fat and needed to lose weight. Growing up, she struggled with her weight which sometimes fluctuated up to 60 pounds in one year. By the time Raquel reached college, she had full-blown eating disorders. She tried any and every diet available, used illegal drugs such as amphetamine, and took extreme measures including bulimia.*

*After years of coping with her own weight challenges, Raquel learned to stop the struggle with addictions, guilt, and poor body image. She experienced a transformation in which she changed her relationship with food and stabilized her weight by aiming to resolve the underlying issues. Raquel now helps others learn how to deal with emotional eating so they can release their weight and transform their lives.*

**Dr. Leyla: What was your life like when you were growing up?**
Raquel: When I was young I was already very aware of my body and weight. For gymnastics, I was supposed to lose three pounds of water weight with each five-hour workout. My weight was constantly monitored and I was often told I was too fat and needed to lose weight. This experience led to a two-decade-long struggle of obsessive-compulsive behavior with dieting.

**Dr. Leyla: How was your family health?**
Raquel: My dad was compulsive overeater and a binge eater. However, he was able to keep his weight under control until he reached his 40s. He ate cartons of ice cream, and he ate in the middle of the night. Everyone knew what he was doing but nobody could help him.

Even after heart surgery and several heart attacks my dad still wasn't able to change. He continued to eat fast food. He died as a morbidly obese man. It was painful for me to watch him deteriorate all the while knowing there was nothing I could do to help.

**Dr. Leyla: How did his eating habits affect you?**
Raquel: At the time, it felt he loved food more than his family. Yet that's an old thought. A doctor told my dad if he "didn't change his life he would die"—yet he couldn't stop. It was a compulsion. This was a big motivator for me to search for the deeper meaning behind compulsions.

**Dr. Leyla: How is your mother's health?**
Raquel: My mother was a health fanatic; ahead of the times. She frequented health food stores, ate carob, grape nuts, and raw foods. She was a renegade.

**Dr. Leyla: How was your weight in high school?**
Raquel: In high school I took benazeprine which is a speed-like diet pill. Even though I was very active, I was never able to reach a comfortable goal weight and maintain. It was always a struggle.

**Dr. Leyla: How was your weight in college?**
Raquel: By the time I was in college, I had full-blown eating disorders. I was a professional dancer, always in good shape, but that made my eating disorder even worse. I never had a dancer's body, and I never looked like a gymnast; I had more of a naturally round body shape. The weight fluctuations often were extreme—sometimes 60 pounds in one year. I would go from 90 pounds to 165 pounds. I often bounced back and forth from being too skinny and emaciated, to being overweight.

**Dr. Leyla: What kind of diets did you try?**
Raquel: I tried Jenny Craig, Nutrisystem, diet pills, no-carb diets, Atkins, watermelon diet, Slim Fast, Pritkin Diet, smoking cigarettes to curb

**102**

my appetite, as well as amphetamines, speed, cocaine, and other drugs to help deal with my food addiction.

**Dr. Leyla: How did your struggle progress after college?**
Raquel: In my late 20s, I started my own dance company, and I had a successful performance group. The money was very good as I had sold-out performances. However, I was managing my weight through cigarettes and amphetamines. I still struggled with compulsive overeating and binging. I was in a lot of emotional pain due to my body image issues and eating disorders.

**Dr. Leyla: When did your transformation take place?**
Raquel: The point where things shifted is when I had a horrible breakup and I lost 50 pounds. I then began eating out of control. One day my binging got to the point where I ended up collapsing on the street corner in tears. This is when I heard this faint little voice that cried "You're hurting me!" At that point, I realized I needed to relearn my relationship to my body and to food. I was feeling out of control, and I had the insight that I was really hurting myself, and it was time to change. I started to become aware that my health and well-being were more important than anything else.

**Dr. Leyla: So what did you do?**
Raquel: I decided to do my own transformational journey. I traveled to a variety of places, including Rome, Egypt, Israel, Mexico, and Peru. I studied with spiritual teachers I met along the way. When I came home I went back to school and got my master's degree in spiritual psychology from the University of Santa Monica.

**Dr. Leyla: Did you plan your trip?**
Raquel: No, I went on a journey with the intention to find my purpose and cross paths with people on the way. I met people who I learned from and who helped me transform and change my path.

**Dr. Leyla: What did you learn about yourself?**
Raquel: I learned that I wasn't longing for food. I was longing for spiritual

connection. I didn't want food as it was just a quick fix. Instead, I wanted to be alive, and to learn how to feel good. I wanted love and to learn to love my body. I realized that my body was a gift from God. I owed it to God to care for my body. I also realized that my body was as precious as the earth itself, and it was disrespectful to abuse it. I saw my drive for the so-called *perfect body* to be superficial and meaningless. It took me many years to understand why we go for things that don't nourish or uplift us. But once I found this awareness, then everything fell into place.

**Dr. Leyla: How has your weight and life been since?**
Raquel: It wasn't sudden. Every year I get healthier and healthier, and I reach a greater level of health. My body weight stays balanced with no more than three-pound fluctuations.

**Dr. Leyla: How has your life changed?**
Raquel: Mentally, spiritually, physically, and emotionally, I am much better. I'm now living my life's purpose; I'm holding the torch for women who are living trapped by their body images. I feel impassioned as my weight was literally my prison. Lots of women suffer from poor body image—it's a very real issue.

**Dr. Leyla: How has your path in life changed?**
Raquel: I started my own business to help women with self-image, and relationship with food. It's not about weight loss; it's really about transforming one's body image.

**Dr. Leyla: What kind of clients do you help?**
Raquel: A lot of my clients had previously asked their medical doctors for help to lose weight. The first thing these doctors are now recommending—even for young women in their 20's—is the gastric bypass surgery. I am horrified by this and what it does to these poor women. Not only does it make them unable to absorb nutrients for their hair, skin, organs, for the rest of their lives, but many gain the weight back within a couple of years. This is because the underlying issues have not been resolved. It is truly so saddening we are dealing with

this cultural crisis in a way that causes more pain, more struggle, and greater illness.

**Dr. Leyla: Why are so many people struggling with their weight?**
Raquel: I now clearly see the obesity epidemic in this country as a cry for help. We are starving internally and we, as a culture, are looking to connect to something deeper than just modern-day consumerism. This country is not having a food crisis or a health crisis; it is having a spiritual crisis. People are calling for a deeper connection and union to their own bodies, to the earth, and to God. We long for greater expressions of love, creativity, and meaning, and it's time to find and create those expressions.

**Dr. Leyla: What is involved in helping people reach their goal?**
Raquel: Primarily I aim to help them discover where they don't value themselves. It's about self-worth, and learning why people do things that hurt themselves. There are things that have happened in our childhoods that we may feel angry about and are not healed. Those places inside that say "you'll never achieve that", "you're not good enough for that." It's not about putting a regimen together to create a diet and exercise plan. It's about creating a need to inspire the desire for health, which comes from a sense of self-worth.

**Dr. Leyla: What kind of programs do you offer?**
Raquel: I offer one day workshops, one-on-one therapy, and I'm also in the process of creating a home-study course. I also put together The New Beauty Revolution with 17 speakers, including Marianne Williamson and David Woolf. The seminar focused on emotional eating and body image.

**Dr. Leyla: What is your greatest success story?**
Raquel: I feel most moved when I help others transform their obsessions with food. Weighing themselves day in and day out, obsessed with what they are going to eat, counting calories, restricting and then binging is horribly painful way to live. I feel fulfilled and successful as I watch women free themselves from this obsession and then have

enough energy to live their life purposes and fulfill their dreams.

**Dr. Leyla: What are your future goals?**
Raquel: To continue to serve on a deeper level. My business has exploded over the past couple months. My goal is to bring my message to more people.

**Dr. Leyla: What message do you want to give to the world?**
Raquel: Set a high intention for healing, rather than just changing your body. The greatest investment you can make is in your health and healing, and being in line with a healthy body. I am truly committed to changing the way women diet and see their bodies. As we express ourselves by fully living, creating, and enjoying life—and by eating more consciously—we will live more healthily. This allows our physical beings to come into alignment with our true divine natures and connections to God. And the best part is our natural beauty will shine through!

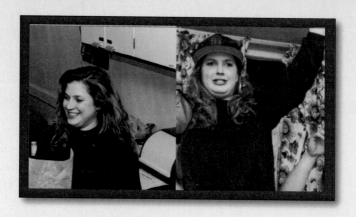

Raquel@endthedietwar.com
(562) 433-6081

EndTheDietWar.com

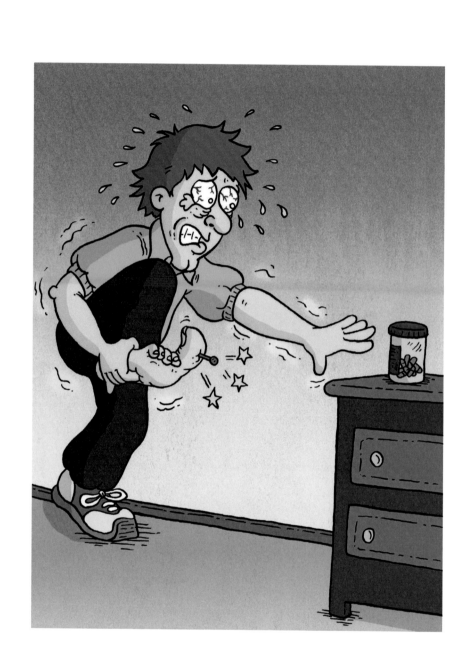

# CHAPTER 7

# PAIN

*Pain is inevitable, Suffering is optional.*
*~Buddhist proverb*

Everyone has experienced some sort of pain. Pain has two purposes: to keep the body in balance, and as a warning sign something is wrong.

There are many people who suffer from some type of chronic pain. At the pharmacy, patients who come for pain medications often become regular, long-term customers. They are demanding and never skip a refill. Yet suffering in pain for so long can often cause people to become mean, bitter, depressed, or angry.

## MEDICAL DOCTOR DIAGNOSIS

A medical doctor will diagnose a patient first by determining the location of the pain. Is it joint pain, nerve pain, muscle pain, or chest pain? The patient describes the pain, as there are several types of pain, including come and go, chronic, stabbing, throbbing, sharp, dull, and constant.[94]

The treatment for pain starts simply:[95]

- First are the low-dose, over-the-counter analgesics, such as ibuprofen (200 mg) and naproxen (220 mg).
- More severe pain will be dealt with by giving higher, prescription-strength doses of these analgesics such as ibuprofen (800 mg) or naproxen (500 mg), which reduces swelling by creating an anti-inflammatory effect.

- Corticosteroids, like prednisone also reduce swelling and are prescribed when other anti-inflammatories either don't work well enough or cause too many side effects. Corticosteroids work by suppressing the immune system.
- Finally there are the opioids such as hydrocodone, oxycontin, and morphine. These narcotics provide stronger pain relief and are addictive.

There are also pain clinics in which doctors will attempt to manage pain by having the patient take regular medication with scheduled doses taken around the clock and possibly another medication for the "breakthrough pain" when the regular pain medication isn't enough.

This is the training provided to the doctors and pharmacists. Their standard education will provide information about types of pain, drugs, more drugs, and higher doses of drugs, and then surgery. There are many doctors that use other types of devices for pain treatment, but generally these are not taught in the standard medical education.

Patients often need medications that are narcotics, such as hydrocodone, oxycontin, or morphine. These are controlled and addictive substances. Over time patients develop a tolerance to a dose of a drug, and will eventually need a higher dose to achieve the same pain relief. Once they start to increase the doses, they get more side effects. Then if the patient loses the pills, or they are in more severe pain and take more than prescribed, they must then request an early refill from the pharmacy. These cases will be documented and often met with suspicion.

Being in pain often leads to other problems as well. All medications have side effects.

- If a patient feels they may not get enough pain medication, they can become anxious.
- Pain sufferers often become depressed[96], especially if their doctors have given them a grim or hopeless diagnosis.
- Long term use of anti-inflammatories can cause ulcers.[97]
- Steroidal anti-inflammatories suppress the immune system leading the patient to become vulnerable to other problems

and diseases.[98]
- Narcotic pain medications cause constipation and higher doses can cause respiratory depression.[99]

The most profitable customers are those who are regular healthcare consumers with no permanent solution in sight, such as those with chronic pain. Often the patients must spend a significant amount of time and energy at the doctors' offices, pharmacies, and dealing with insurance companies. This can be time consuming and emotionally exhausting, affecting their quality of life.

## ALTERNATIVE TREATMENTS FOR PAIN

Unfortunately, often patients don't seek alternatives until the medical system has failed them, and they've been suffering for years. Still, there are several ways to address pain rather than drugs and surgery. As I have explored the world of alternative health, I have met several people who have suffered for YEARS after a poor or even hopeless prognosis by their doctor, only to find pain relief from alternative means. Art San's story in the back of the chapter is one example.

Here are some examples of different ways to deal with pain from an alternative or holistic perspective.

**Stress and Emotions.** Poorly handled or excess stress can lead to a physical manifestation of pain. Medical doctors may or may not acknowledge this connection. Holistically, pain is another expression that something is off balance. There are some various ways to deal with emotions, such as Somatic Trauma Resolution, and Emotional Freedom Technique.[100]

**Meditation.**[101] This teaches people how to train the mind to induce a mode of consciousness using deep slow breathing. Meditation has been used to help pain patients control their mind and thus reduce their pain.

**Yoga.** Associated with meditation, it combines the power of the mind with stretching, which can help reduce pain.

**Acupuncture.**[102] According to Traditional Chinese Medicine, all types of pain are caused by blockage of energy. Inserting and manipulating needles into the various acupuncture points can release the energy blockage and relieve the pain.

**Pain is Energy–Dahn Yoga.**[103] In this unique Korean yoga form, one practice is to sit in a pose for an extended period of time. For example, the practitioner might lie on his or her back, with the legs and hands in the air, for from 5 to 20 minutes. At some point there is pain in the legs or another part of the body. By continuing the pose, one can feel the pain, or energy, moving up the leg and being released.

**Biofeedback.**[104] This is an instrument that reads the physiological function of the body and attempts to make adjustments. Biofeedback can train a patient to interact with their brain so his or her brain reads pain differently, causing the patient to feel less pain.

**Hypnotherapy.** Our subconscious mind runs our body. Hypnosis is a method in which you give explicit commands to the subconscious mind that can be used to relieve pain, among many other health conditions or reasons.

**Health Opportunity.** According to some holistic practices, any health condition is actually a health opportunity, where one has the opportunity to grow and learn and to become closer to the spiritual and true self. What do I need to learn from this pain? What are the good things that have happened as a result of this pain?

## LONG-TERM CUSTOMERS WITH SHORT-TERM RELIEF

Current medical practice has a well-defined set of *solutions* that have become the most popular often because they are the best business system.

**112**

These methods of pain relief create **long-term customers with short-term relief,** creating the vicious cycle of temporary relief and permanent customers. Because our human response is often accepting that *doctor knows best,* many become slaves to pharmaceuticals, believing it is the best or only option.

There are often better solutions to pain. But the standard medical doctor is not trained in these various modalities. Therefore, a patient must take responsibility to research the different types of alternative treatments available.

**POINTS TO REMEMBER:**

- Patients who suffer from chronic pain often create long-term profit for doctors and pharmacies.

- There are many who have suffered with so-called incurable conditions or pain that has been treated successfully by alternative or holistic approaches.

## INTERVIEW WITH SPORTS MASSAGE THERAPIST ART SAN

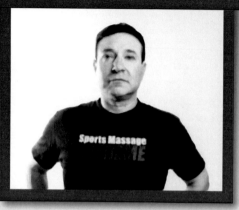

*Art San was a social worker when he got in a motorcycle accident that led him to be in severe back pain for over 20 years. He was unable to jump, run, or lie down for extended periods of time. Medical doctors offered a poor prognosis and Art refused surgery. When Art was at a swap meet, he saw a massage tool for 75 cents that he intuitively knew would get him out of pain. Using a combination of pressure points and massage therapy, Art was able to finally alleviate his pain and misery.*

*Art is now a massage therapist who created his own special technique to help treat others. He spends his time working as "The Pain Eraser", helping people who have received a poor prognosis from the doctors, and those who have accepted pain, tightness, and discomfort as part of their lives.*

**Dr. Leyla: Tell me about your accident.**
Art San: I was in a motorcycle accident, where I injured my lower back, fracturing my vertebrae at the L4 and L5, among other injuries.

**Dr. Leyla: How did the medical doctors treat your pain?**
Art San: I had just turned 20 years old and my doctor told me that I should expect to have chronic back problems and pain for the rest of my life. I wore a plaster cast on both my chest and leg for several months.

**Dr. Leyla: Did you take pain medications?**
Art San: I refused prescription narcotics, as I was in a place in my life where I chose to be drug and alcohol free. My doctor told me to take Tylenol three times per day because that might provide some relief.

**Dr. Leyla: What treatments did you attempt, in order to manage the pain?**
Art San: I tried acupuncture and a few different chiropractors. Nothing worked.

**Dr. Leyla: What was your life like during those years of chronic pain?**
Art San: It was really tough. I would have to wake up extra early just to stretch out. I couldn't lie in bed for more than 15 to 20 minutes without suffering later in the day. I couldn't sit still for longer than 30 minutes without fidgeting—to avoid severe lower back spasms and cramps. I couldn't run or jump, and I had muscle spasms and cramping every day, several times throughout the day. Worst of all, for years I accepted what the doctor had told me and I believed that this was how my life was going to be.

**Dr. Leyla: How did you finally relieve your pain?**
Art San: Actually, I was at a swap meet when I saw this certain massage tool. I wasn't looking for ways to treat my pain—I didn't think it was possible. But when I saw this tool, I knew instantly that it was going to somehow give me the relief I needed. Intuitively, I knew how to use it. So I bought it, went home, and started to experiment. By combining use of the tool with my basic massage therapy training, I was able to get myself out of pain within a week.

**Dr. Leyla: What is your background?**
Art San: For 15 years, I worked as a certified substance abuse counselor, and then as a program coordinator and trainer. After that I worked as an assistant sales director. Currently, I am the founder of Sports Massage Extreme of Los Angeles, CA.

**Dr. Leyla: What is the theory behind your technique?**
Art San: To summarize, after an injury, the muscles in your body tighten to compensate, in an effort to readjust or realign. It is often this tightening of the muscles that causes much of the inflammation and pain that people feel. My technique involves the releasing of these tight muscles.

**Dr. Leyla: What training did you have to learn this technique?**
Art San: After I relieved myself of pain, I took more advanced massage training and learned reflexology. I created this technique. It is basically a combination of reflexology and massage. I also incorporate trigger points and some myofascial release.

**Dr. Leyla: Why do you think so many people are suffering in pain?**
Art San: In my opinion, there are two major contributing factors. First the overall stress level (of the population) is much higher than it was 20 years ago. Second, people have increased their use and reliance on pharmaceutical drugs. These days, patients in pain expect a doctor or pill to solve their problems; many folks have simply stopped looking within themselves for solutions.

**Dr. Leyla: What type of pain does your technique work with?**
Art San: Migraines, Temporomandibular Joint disorders (TMJ), frozen shoulder, tennis and golf injuries, carpel tunnel syndrome, plantar fascitis, nerve pain, and back pain, to name a few.

**Dr. Leyla: Many people don't have significant pain but have muscles that are extremely tight and inflexible as they get older. Do you also help with tightness and flexibility?**
Art San: Absolutely. I help athletes maintain their flexibility. I also help accident victims and others regain their range of motion. Many people lose a lot of flexibility, and work around their tight muscles by walking differently or by adjusting their movements to avoid pain. If not corrected, these adjustments will keep your body progressing on the wrong track and can lead to more pain and more problems. I've also helped diabetic patients with neuropathy, and stroke patients regain feeling.

**Dr. Leyla: How can people learn these techniques themselves?**
Art San: When I work on a person, I give them the knowledge and the tools to continue their own treatment. I will also be holding training sessions in the future so other practitioners can learn and share this technique as well.

**Dr. Leyla: How is your life today?**
Art San: Happy, free, full of energy. I always enjoy great sleep. After twenty years of not being able to lie down for more than 20 minutes, you can't imagine how much I appreciate a night's rest. So many people are fortunate, and take this seemingly innocuous event for granted. Today, I can stay in bed for eight hours with no cramping whatsoever. I also do my self-applied maintenance routine daily to keep myself pain free.

**Dr. Leyla: How rewarding is your work?**
Art San: I feel truly blessed to be able to share this gift with others. To treat someone in pain who, like me, had given up hope of ever moving without discomfort, is the most rewarding gift I could hope for and truly keeps me motivated every day.

**Art San**
**Sports Massage Extreme**
**643 South Olive Street, Suite 830**
**Los Angeles, CA 90014**
**(310) 753-2276**

**SportsMassageExtreme.com**

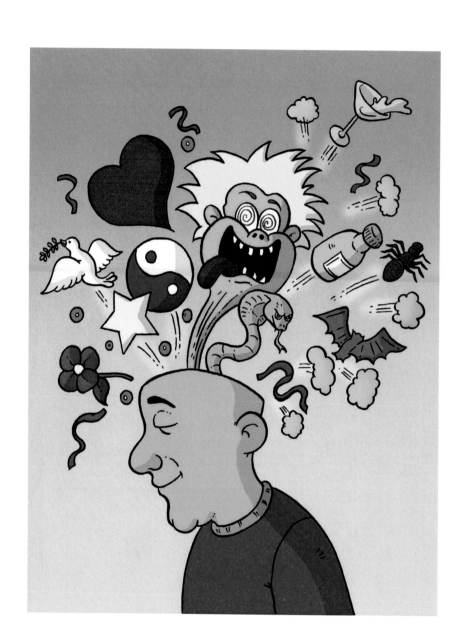

# CHAPTER 8

# POWER OF THE MIND

*You have the power to heal your life, and you need to know that. We think so often that we are helpless, but we're not. We always have the power of our minds…Claim and consciously use your power.*
*~Louise L Hay*

When I applied for pharmacy school, I felt I was prepared for the challenge. I had completed my bachelor's degree in anthropology, and then I had taken two more years of classes to prepare me for pharmacy school, including chemistry, biology, and physics. I had a respectable grade-point average and worked part-time in a pharmacy. The pharmacists who I worked with told me I'd have no problem getting accepted. So when the interview process came along, I didn't prepare for it as well as I should have. As a result, I was put on the wait list for both schools to which I had applied.

But I had made up my mind to go. I had nothing else I needed to do; I took all the required courses and I had no back-up plan. I called both schools often to touch base and to check the status of the wait list. The employee that I spoke with at one of the schools was not very helpful, the other was friendlier.

As the months passed and the beginning of school was getting closer, I called more consistently. I was getting nervous, but at the same time I imagined the feeling of being accepted. It was now Friday, and classes started the next week. I called and the friendly lady that I normally spoke with wasn't in. I sat in silence for a moment as my heart dropped with hope fading.

**119**

She continued "She should be in a little later. Would you like to leave a message?"

"Yes" I replied, "Can you please tell her that my bags are packed and I'm ready to go."

On Monday she called back. I was at work.

"Are you sure you're ready?"

"YES, I'm ready!"

That day a friend came along for the five-hour drive. He bought my books and found an apartment for me while I started the first day of classes.

That is the power of the mind. I imagined it. I was focused on it. I needed to go. I had nothing else to do. And I felt that I deserved to go. Although at that time I didn't even realize what powers I was tapping into.


## THE MIND

The mind is so powerful, it can drive us crazy, or keep us in denial, energize happiness and bliss, or solve mathematical and relationship problems. It instantaneously absorbs and defines what we see, feel, hear, taste, touch, and smell. In school, our minds are trained to listen, read, memorize, write, solve math problems, and imagine. However, the mind has powers that we don't learn about in school, which many never learn about, and therefore will never tap into.

The mind has the power to create the circumstances in our lives. If properly trained, it has the power to heal the body. In terms of wellness, humans have amazing capabilities to self-heal, or mend, unhealthy attitudes and habits.

Unfortunately, there is not much profit in making others aware of how powerful the mind can be. Therefore this truth is not well promoted in today's society of quick fixes and immediate pain relief. Instead of empowering the population to use their natural abilities at the highest level, the pharmaceutical companies create a need and demand for their product in the name of profit. The American population has been dumbed-down to the point that truth is sourced via repetitive advertising and sound bites—the scale and depth of this travesty is only now being revealed. Advertisers understand how to appeal to the emotions and make the mind believe or feel something that will lead them to more profits. We have, both voluntarily and involuntarily, given up control of our thoughts, feelings and emotions. Many industries—food, auto, housing and banking to name a few—have capitalized on this. They ring up profits and fortunes in the process. No business has done a better and more damaging job of this than pharmaceutical companies. They create and sell solutions to our illnesses before we even know we suffer. It has completely replaced the healing power of the mind, individually and collectively.

## CREATING A HYPE

One summer, I traveled to England with my father. We were doing the tourist thing on a bustling London street when, suddenly, a gentleman placed his briefcase on the sidewalk and opened it up. Almost immediately, a crowd gathered around, as he barked, "Gold for Sale! Gold for Sale!" I couldn't see what was going on, so I squeezed in for a look. To my amazement, people were holding out money, just waiting for their turn to get the seller's attention and make a purchase. My eyes lit up when I saw all that gold; I watched in awe. Then, a lady with an English accent turned to me and said, "It's a really good buy, you know." I was sold, and I slipped back to discuss with my father, "Should we get some?" I asked excitedly.

He was chuckling good-naturedly. "Let's just watch for a while." We stepped aside and observed for about twenty minutes. The woman who told me, "It's a good buy," proceeded to make a purchase, then moved about ten feet away, where she lingered for about five minutes before diving back into the mix of people. Interestingly—shockingly to me, but not my father—she bought more. As we continued to observe we watched as others in the group repeated the same pattern as that woman, creating the hype in order to attract passersby. In total, there were about eight people involved in the show. Finally, my father was laughing so much that

**121**

he was disturbing their system, or façade, and he was confronted by one of the players who suggested we move along.

This was my very first lesson in the art of creating hype. My father explained afterwards that people are easily influenced. The human species has evolved to the point that we want a good deal, we want it now, and we want it cheaply. Since that time in London, I've always been aware of the possibility that if "it's too good to be true," then it often is. Granted, I can still get suckered, but it's with eyes wide open. I am always thankful for that London street learning experience.

At the same time, there is an art and technique to creating hype. Good advertisers know how to create a demand for their product, making the masses want or even better, *need* their product. They understand how to appeal to the emotions, and make their wares look sexy and desirable. Cigarettes are a great example. Logically, they're expensive, toxic, cause cancer, stink, and have no features that make them a worthy purchase. There's the lady in public service commercials who continues to smoke through the tracheotomy hole in her throat.[105] Despite the fact that the tobacco caused cancer, she's still addicted. However, people still smoke, and teenagers are continuing to start smoking. It has a carefree, sexy, rebellious appeal. By the time that smokers figure out that it's not so sexy, it's too late; they're addicted.

## PLACEBO EFFECT

Drug companies know the power of the mind, and over decades have perfected the process and framework to profit from this awareness. The development stage of any new drug involves research, testing and FDA approval. First the problem is identified, or created, and then a drug is introduced. Extensive trial periods provide information in order to tweak a drug's intent and side effects. Here lies proof that pill producers know the mind's strength in influencing human endeavors. How else could the use of placebo be developed into an art form?

A placebo is defined as:

*A substance with no pharmacological effect but administered as a control in testing, experimentally or clinically, the efficacy of a biologically active preparation.*[106]

So, in order to evaluate a drug's potential value, or marketability, the pharmaceutical companies must test its effectiveness by comparing it to a sugar pill, a fake.

The placebo effect is defined as:

*A reaction to a placebo manifested by a lessening of symptoms or the production of anticipated side effects. The placebo effect occurs when a patient receives an expected effect from the drug, even though there is no drug, or pharmacologically active agent, within the pill.*[107]

In other words, by simply telling a patient they're ingesting helpful medication, test administrators cause patients' bodies to manifest relief. There are several cases where the placebo produced better equal or better results than the tested drug![108]  In controlled clinical trials, the patients who took placebos, with no active drug, got better results than those taking the drug being tested.  The studies must take the placebo effect into consideration because researchers know the mind has the power to heal.


## LAW OF ATTRACTION

Whatever you focus upon creates your reality.  If you focus on positive things, then you get positive experiences.  If you focus on the negative things, you get negative experiences.[109]

One method used to help create a reality is affirmations, in which you speak and focus on your desires.  Through the power of imagination and visualization you can let yourself see, feel, taste, smell, and touch your desires and the world you want to create.

The subconscious mind is tricky.  It does not understand negatives.  If you focus on what you don't want to become, then you will create that which you don't want.  In other words, if you create an affirmation "I am healthy and energetic" then that's what your subconscious mind will understand and work to create. However, if you do affirmations of "I want to prevent cancer", according to your subconscious mind, you are focusing on cancer and will actually be attracting cancer.

In our world most of the voices and messages we hear are not our own affirmations, but messages from advertisers, telling us how to prevent this or that. Besides putting the thought of the condition or disease in our minds, they are also putting their proposed solution and product in as well. Suddenly much of the population is focused on whatever the drug companies can profit from and therefore wish to advertise. As a result, those with the most money create the advertisements, the affirmations, which often eventually become our realities—if we let them.

To further this, often we say things in passing, that if repeated over and over, the subconscious mind will believe and eventually create. We say things like "I'm falling apart" or "I'm afraid of being happy because something bad always happens." Often people make these types of comments in passing, not realizing how powerful and potentially harmful they can be.

## BELIEF SYSTEM

Our human evolution embraced many ideas, or beliefs, that were, at the time, considered undeniable truths. These were founding principles or beliefs that lasted for generations. It wasn't until discovered otherwise, for example, that all people believed:

- The world was flat, and the edge was treacherous.
- The earth was the center of all existence.

Science, underlying curiosity, and eventually human experience bring the mind to greater understanding of "what is." Consider certain mindsets that permeated more recent belief systems, which were reflected in laws of the land:

- Native Americans were savages. Therefore, it was okay to exact violence upon them.

**124**

- Black people, brought to America as slaves, were considered property, not fellow humans.
- Women were inferior to men, and should not have the right to vote.

As the world evolved and matured, so did the recognition that certain laws were not only outdated, but outright wrong, and needed to be abolished.

If we go back to cigarettes, for example: it's amazing to consider that, for decades, smoking cigarettes was not considered to be a risk. Even with the non-refutable scientific linkage between smoke inhalation and lung damage, *cancer sticks* continued to be promoted as *sexy*. Everybody who was anybody smoked. It was cool. Our belief systems do not go away easily, and usually significant pain and suffering is the only catalyst to change our beliefs.

Think about certain American standards of living, especially the labels placed on them. Cotton swabs are Q-tips and tissues are Kleenex. Why is that? Advertising is a phenomenon of epic proportions in our society that directly impacts how people think, feel, and what they believe. The mind has been trained and programmed to consider what it sees and hears to be the truth. Advertisers know this, which is why the modern understanding of truth is slanted by the delivery of the message. Our society is inundated with messages and information powered by ulterior motives, from WebMD to drug commercials, as they quickly mumble the lengthy list of side effects and disclaimers inherent in prescription medicine advertisements.

WebMD, with their loads of information, has established itself as the gold standard for trusted healthcare information in our society. Yet in reality it is also an extremely biased tool to promote the pharmaceutical industry. Notice their discussion of cancer treatment:

*"Cancer treatment includes chemotherapy, radiation, and surgery. If you're considering complementary treatments for cancer, discuss this with your doctor as they may interact with other cancer treatment."* [110]

**125**

"If you're considering complementary treatments . . . may interact with other cancer treatments". Of course, nobody wants anything natural to interfere with the toxic chemotherapy! But notice how the words subtly discredit the complementary medicine, almost suggesting that it gets in the way of the real treatment and potentially causes problems.

This type of language is seen all over WebMD, the most trusted, yet biased, website available for drug companies. It's promoted as complete health information resource, yet the expertise that they hold is in the promotion of doctors and drugs. This is another reminder that doctors have become experts on drugs, not health.

## ANATOMY OF DRUG COMMERCIAL

We've all seen the commercials that practically saturate the media:

- Appeal to the emotions.
- Create curiosity and how to offer hope.
- A technique the drug companies use to gain trust and create more profits.

Consider the standard formula for a commercial:

1. Show the symptoms of a health condition or disease:

   - Present a stressed out person, experiencing sadness, anxiety, high cholesterol.
   - Identify the health condition by name: depression, Alzheimer's, high cholesterol, etc.
   - Elicit sympathy for the person, who will be likeable yet suffering, and worthy of the viewer's concern.

2. Then introduce a drug. The screen changes from black and white to color and the person's days get brighter.

3. Side effects are mentioned in a quieter, rapid tone in one big sentence with images of happy experiences that do not match. Show people doing

happy, fun things that are completely unrelated, like walking on an exotic beach, strolling through a beautiful garden, or cheering at an exciting sports event.

Only seven percent of communication is created through words. Visual communication accounts for 55 percent, and tone is 38 percent. Therefore, the images on the screen are much more powerful than any spoken words. And since the tone is 38 percent, speaking in a fast, quieter, monotone ensures much less will be heard or retained.[111]

Imagine if the drug companies were forced to give visual images that matched the words. When they listed the side effects, they would have to actually show people experiencing them. What would happen to drug sales if liver damage was a side effect of the drug? The commercials would therefore have to show a man unconscious in a hospital bed, surrounded by his worried wife and children, and then display his name on the waiting list for a liver.

4. Call to action: "Ask your doctor if this drug is right for you."

In the past, pharmaceutical companies were only allowed to advertise to medical doctors, who knew what was best for the patient and would make the decision about what to prescribe. However, in 1997 the direct-to-consumer advertising laws were changed, allowing pharmaceutical companies to advertise straight to the population.[112] Imagine the increase in sales now that patients are coming into a doctor's office and requesting a medication. According to surveys, when a patient requests a specific drug, 70 percent of the time the doctors will write a prescription for the patient's request.[113]

## PAST MEDICAL BELIEFS

In the past, there were several procedures that where common, or standard practice by the professionals. Today, we look back at them as ludicrous.

For example:
- A procedure called bloodletting was a popular medical practice.[114]

When a patient was sick the standard procedure would be bleed out an amount of blood to cure the imbalance of fluids in the body.
- In the 1920s women took capsules filled with tapeworm eggs to lose weight.[115]
- There was also a procedure called trepanation, or drilling a hole in the head, which was used to treat seizures and migraines.[116]

These extreme and completely ridiculous procedures were recommended by the experts of the time, and became the reality of the time. In fact, there were several standard practices that happened in the past but seem completely ludicrous today. Will people look back at this time with similar disbelief? In one hundred years from now (or hopefully sooner) the history books will speak of a time when the masses considered doctors as authority and their words as fact, as patients took pill after pill and expected improvements in their health. Meanwhile they suffered for years with conditions that often could be easily treated by holistic healthcare practitioners. Will future generations laugh and call the people of our time *ignorant* or *primitive*?

## MODERN DOCTOR'S AND PHARMACIST'S FALSE BELIEFS

Here are a few more blatant and painful examples of skewed messages being absorbed by the mind:

- Just ask your doctor or pharmacist.
- Pharmacists consistently rank as one of the most trusted professions.
- Your condition is "incurable."
- Doctors are experts on our health.

We the people give over our health and wellness to the doctors and pharmacists, who have the trusted role in our society and are expected to know and understand our health better than ourselves. However, they have been filled with knowledge by the major manufacturers of pills. The profits created by their work are used to create mega-advertising which gives them even more exposure and credibility that works to maintain the

**128**

façade. Drug companies know too well the intricacies of influencing the mind. Yet they use that knowledge to create repeat customers and more profits, rather than better health.

## BABY ELEPHANT SYNDROME

There is a story about a baby elephant who is tied to a tree by a heavy chain. The baby elephant thrashes around with all his might to get free, but he cannot as he is not strong enough. So eventually he gives up. When the elephant grows up and is much stronger, he can then be tied by a thin rope to a small tree and he will not try to get away. His mind has been conditioned by its prior experiences, so he doesn't make the slightest attempt to break free. Even though the elephant has plenty of strength to get free, he doesn't know that and therefore no longer tries. The large and powerful elephant has limited its present abilities based on the limitations learned in the past.

We rely on doctors to give a diagnosis and prognosis and we rely on them to tell us what's possible or not possible with our healing and health. Human beings are very similar to the struggling elephant, as once limitations are set, it is hard to move past them. However, we can choose not to accept false boundaries and limitations of our past and of the medical profession.

## *WHAT CAN WE DO ABOUT IT?*

With all the bad and unhealthy information provided to us these days, what is the answer? How can a person move forward, discover truth, and retrain the mind into more positive territory? How can one tap into and take control of the power of the mind?

## TAKING BACK CONTROL OF OUR MINDS

**Tune It Out.** The first step in regaining control of our thoughts is tuning out useless, negative information like television advertisements. There's lots of noise out there, whether it's television or conversations with friends. If it doesn't serve you and only adds bad information or feelings, tune it out.

Much information is absorbed by our minds at a subconscious level. Turn off the images and commercials that affect the mind. Turn off the news completely. Watching the news used to be a sign of intelligence, of being informed. But do you really have to see every negative thing that happened, every murder, rape, or celebrity scandal? Watch the news and notice how much of the information is educational, relevant or important to know. Then notice how much is junk. Most of it is bad news and not necessary information for our lives. Be extremely picky about the information that you listen to and are open to.

**Thoughts.** Similarly, create awareness about your thoughts and be picky with what you allow into your head. Although it may take some training and practice, we can choose our thoughts and our beliefs. Once you identify a negative thought, you can choose to change your perspective and create better thoughts. Again, this is a practice, but it can be a very useful and powerful habit to create.

**Expand Your Thoughts and Beliefs.** Do you believe that your mind has the potential to create and heal more than most can imagine? Unfortunately, the powers of our minds are often exploited by drug companies and others that can make a profit. There are no big bucks to be made by a company that tells you that you can heal on your own, or teaches you how to empower yourself. Again, the profits come when a company convinces you that you need them or their product to maintain good health.

In fact, our bodies have healed by themselves for years. It is only in the past century that drugs have become standard or necessary. Yet we have come so far away from the basics, and the messages from advertisers are so ingrained in our vulnerable and open minds. Question your own beliefs, from the small to the large. Is this true? Are there other possibilities? For example, some people believe they will get the flu every winter. Is this true? Does it need to be?

**130**

**Visualization.** Our most underutilized resource is our own imagination, where we can create worlds. This is the secret and magic of the universe that most don't know about. If we use our minds to create images in which we can actually feel the sensations of our creations, we can learn to intentionally create our realities.

**Healing With Visualization.** You can heal yourself with your mind. Some people have destroyed cancer by the power of their minds and visualization. Please note interview with Susan H Moss at the end of chapter 10. Also check out Duncan Tooley's healing journey using hypnotherapy at the end of this chapter. Additionally, Wayne Dyer is a teacher of this method.[117]

## CHECK IT OUT

My favorite people who teach expanding your thoughts are:

- Success coach Tony Robbins, who shows how to change, expand and succeed.
- When it comes to health, author Louise Hay's book "You Can Heal Your Life" offers new thought patterns for health and the possibility to heal oneself from conditions deemed incurable by medical doctors.
- Mike Dooley, author of "Infinite Possibilities,"[118] has a CD on expanding your beliefs.

## THE MIND IS POWERFUL

Will you believe the commercials that are specializing in capturing the emotions and creating a demand for their product? Or will you use your mind to empower yourself and to heal?

## POINTS TO REMEMBER:

- Our minds have the power to heal.

- The pharmaceutical companies understand this power of the mind, yet they use their knowledge to create demand, dependency, and profit.

- We need to take control and learn how to use the power of our minds for our own benefit.

## INTERVIEW WITH HYPNOTHERAPIST
## DUNCAN TOOLEY

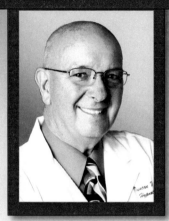

*Duncan Tooley, a former computer programmer and systems analyst for 35 years, suffered from neuropathy so badly that he would fall down when he walked. His work put him on disability and his doctors told him there was nothing they could do for the nerve loss so they gave him drugs to help with his pain. They also put him on a biweekly hospital infusion to lessen his symptoms from the autoimmune damage. He then joined his wife in a hypnotherapy class intending to improve his stained glass artwork, and came out with techiques on how to treat himself. He has been able to fully heal himself from the neuropathy using hypnotherapy. Duncan now works full time as a hypnotherapist helping others overcome their health obstacles.*

**Dr. Leyla: What was your life like before?**
Duncan: I was a science teacher in a high school where I taught chemistry, mathematics, and physics. Then I took computer programming and from there I worked as a computer programmer, then system analyst. I did computer design and administration in engineering, R&D, five years in Europe and then the Computer Science Corporation. I got to be on the team that specified and installed big payroll and human resource systems for states.

**Dr. Leyla: Generally speaking how was your health?**
Duncan: I was always in good shape physically, except when I ruptured a disc in my spine and had surgery. But otherwise I had no problems until the neuropathy set in.

**Dr. Leyla: What was the neuropathy like?**
Duncan: I had peripheral neuropathy so the nerves in my feet, which

are supposed to send signals to the brain through nerve conduction weren't working correctly and were extremely slow. For example, when you step on uneven ground, the feet sense this and normally notify the brain quickly so the body will adjust to compensate and balance itself. But my brain wouldn't be notified until it was too late and I began falling about twice a week. Also there were times when all of a sudden my feet and legs up to my knees would get numb without warning, and then stay numb for a while.

**Dr. Leyla: Is this why you left your job?**
Duncan: My employer required that I go on disability as I could be a liability to them by falling on their client's premises where I was consulting. A year later they just fired me while I was on disability.

**Dr. Leyla: Did you also experience pain with your condition?**
Duncan: Yes, it felt like burning pain. It wasn't too severe but it was constant.

**Dr. Leyla: Do you know why you have this condition?**
Duncan: There are over 250 different types of neuropathy, and often the cause is genetic. The doctors could not identify a specific cause for mine.

**Dr. Leyla: What did the doctors give you to treat it?**
Duncan: The first doctor gave me Neurontin, which is supposed to reduce nerve pain, but it really didn't do much. The doctor would stick me with pins to see if it was getting worse or better. Then once the neuropathy got bad enough he did a nerve biopsy. In this procedure they clip a nerve and make a slide of it. When they cut the nerve it felt like a bolt of lightning.

**Dr. Leyla: What did they find out from that test?**
Duncan: According to the doctor there are two possible causes. The first is nerve sheath damage from an autoimmune condition, in which the immune system attacks the nerve. The second is nerve loss where there are supposed to be a bundle of nerves, but the nerves just aren't there. Without nerves there's not much the doctors can do. I had both types.

**Dr. Leyla: So he had no solution for you?**
Duncan: I took methadone for pain and it helped somewhat, but the drug was controlled. The prescriptions had to be handwritten and picked up each week. It was just too much hassle to get the scripts after a while.

**Dr. Leyla: So then what happened?**
Duncan: I learned of a Methodist Hospital in Houston (in conjunction with Anderson hospital) which had a special neuropathy department. People come from all over the country for their three-day program. So I headed over there.

**Dr. Leyla: Did you get good results?**
Duncan: On the second day there, the doctor who runs the program told me that he thought that he could help me. I received gamma globulin (IVIG), which was to help with the autoimmune portion of the condition that caused the demyelization and damage to the nerve sheaths. Gamma globulin is a blood extract, which has all of the proteins and other components needed to boost the immune system and make it function properly. It's supposed to overpower your immune system and correct the auto immune function. It costs $10,000 per treatment.

**Dr. Leyla: How long did you use that?**
Duncan: I went every two weeks. I had to be in the hospital for 8 hours as it was an infusion and had to be injected over an eight-hour period of time. I did that twice a month for 18 months.

**Dr. Leyla: Did it help?**
Duncan: I could feel that it made a difference. I had more energy, and was feeling better, but then there would be a gradual decline until the time for the next infusion.

**Dr. Leyla: When did you decide to see a hypnotherapist?**
Duncan: My wife Dona reconnected with a friend who was a hypnotherapist. My wife was abused when she was a child, and it was still a problem for her. Yet with one session of hypnotherapy she was able

to face these lifelong abuse issues. So she decided to become a hypnotherapist.

I was still on disability, and spending my time creating stained glass artwork. I would go to the hotel with my wife, talk on the phone, and try to sell my stained glass to architects while she was in a class. She took the course of Shelly Stockwell, who is one of the leading hypnotherapists. I had the pleasure to meet Shelly Stockwell who suggested I become a hypnotherapist too. She said it would make me a better stained glass artist. I wasn't working, so I figured I'd give it a try.

**Dr. Leyla: What did you learn?**
Duncan: In class I heard that the subconscious mind runs our body. It was the first time I heard anything like that. It was interesting, so then I decided to take the second course. Right before the second course I had a case of pink urine. I went to the doctor and he confirmed it was blood. I didn't have time to get it checked as we were about to get on a plane and be gone for 10 days. I had to either miss the class, or wait 10 days until I got back. Instead, I tried the technique used in class: I relaxed and told my subconscious mind "I know you're running my body, I know you know what's wrong. I command you to fix it now."

**Dr. Leyla: So did it work?**
Duncan: The next day the urine was normal color, and it stayed normal. So I didn't go back to the doctor. But then my wife suggested "Why don't you use that on your neuropathy?"

**Dr. Leyla: Once you decided to work on the neuropathy, how long did it take to heal yourself?**
Duncan: It took about five weeks. I ordered the nerves to grow back and I ordered my immune system to leave them alone. I did that every day. I relaxed and gave those commands. Soon I started feeling better. I then stopped taking Neurontin and skipped my infusions. I continued to feel better and better.

**Dr. Leyla: Then did you decide to go back to work in the computer world?**
Duncan: No. What I learned is so powerful that I should have heard about

it before. If I had known about hypnosis back then, I may not have needed surgery for my back. So I decided to change my life and become a hypnotherapist and hypnotherapy instructor. I am now an instructor in the International Hypnosis Federation of which the president is Dr. Shelly Stockwell-Nicholas.

**Dr. Leyla: How does hypnosis work?**
Duncan: Hypnosis is a tool which gets you more in tune with your subconscious and the power that you have because of your connection to the divine. There are lots of stories of spontaneous remission that the experts can't explain. These are people who are using the power of the mind and power of belief to affect the change in their bodies.

**Dr. Leyla: How do you use hypnotherapy in your daily life?**
Duncan: I use self-hypnosis in several ways: whenever I want my attitude to be different, and whenever I don't feel right I use it with the mantra "Every little cell in my body is happy and well."

**Dr. Leyla: What kind of clients do you treat with your hypnotherapy?**
Duncan: Clients come in for weight, anxiety, stress, chronic pain, anxiety about exams, teeth grinding, bedwetting, insomnia, and fears about losing their livelihood. I help people who can't swallow pills. I also helped a guy who kept gagging with his dentures, and a variety of other problems. The possibilities of hypnotherapy are practically limitless. I teach people to use their own power to treat themselves, and that each person has all the power to be, do, and have all that they want.

**Dr. Leyla: Have you used hypnotherapy with your family?**
Duncan: My two daughters practice hypnotherapy as well, and they both used it to have pain-free simple births. Society has pushed women into believing there has to be pain, but it doesn't have to be that way.

**Dr. Leyla: I know you're a follower of Abraham Hicks. How do you explain what their message is about?**
Duncan: Your subconscious mind is running your habits, emotions, body, pretty much your whole life. When you're able to focus and train your

mind, you have much clearer access to all those things. That energy you radiate will be at a different level to attract those things. Abraham Hicks teaches the law of attraction. Whatever you're thinking or feeling, that energy is radiating out to attract others who are thinking or radiating similar thoughts. Your thoughts create your reality.

**Dr. Leyla: How does that incorporate Abraham Hicks' message into your hypnotherapy practice?**
Duncan: I distribute the Hicks CDs. I first convince clients of the importance of what they're thinking—their self-talk. What they want expressed in a positive way that makes them feel good—helps them clear out the negative—is always the start of hypnosis session. If they get that, and they already know or practice it, I ask them if they know about Abraham Hicks.

**Dr. Leyla: Do you believe that anything can be cured with hypnotherapy?**
Duncan: According to Abraham Hicks, there is no body that cannot be made well. Yes, I believe that the power of your belief and getting out of the way of it happening will allow your body to complete its natural movement into balance and wellness.

**Dr. Leyla: Do you have some good success stories?**
Duncan: I had one client come for three sessions for pain. He also had Lyme disease as well as other issues. I gave him an Abraham Hicks CD. He took the information and ran with it. He started getting rid of all his negative thinking and in a matter of days was able to make a fist which he hasn't been able to do for years, and he got rid of his limp. He started moving so rapidly with the law of attraction program that his results were amazing.

**Dr. Leyla: What happens during a hypnotherapy session?**
Duncan: There are a few processes that I often use. One is that I lead the client to their throne where they are filled with grace, light, wisdom and power. They feel the crown on their head, and while in their powerful state they can call for the all-wise and all-knowing part of themselves,

that is connected to divine wisdom of the universe, and ask that part of themselves questions such as "what is holding you back from getting what you want?", and "do you want to release it?" They know the answers and they find and verbalize them. Just about everyone wants to release what is impeding their progress. If they want to hang on, we continue the conversation and find out why. Maybe they're just afraid of change. Eventually they find out what they need to do to get beyond where they are. Then I'll have them take some deep breathes, exhale out of their body and mind whatever is holding them back. They decide what they can do, beginning today, to make progress, and resolve to do it. I give them a post hypnotic suggestion, an anchor, so they can interview their higher self again.

**Dr. Leyla: What is your message to the world?**
Duncan: I was told by a medical expert that there wasn't anything they could do to help my condition. We are often told limitations and what is or isn't possible. My message would be to ask for more and expect more! There is a flow of "Well-Being Energy" that you participate in and that gives you the power over your body. That power is activated by thinking positively and expecting the positive results that you want without concerning yourself that it might be beyond the boundaries of what others believe!

**Duncan Tooley**
**2780 Skypark Drive, Suite 205**
**Torrance, CA  90505**
**(310) 832-0830**

**DuncanTooleyHypnosis.com**

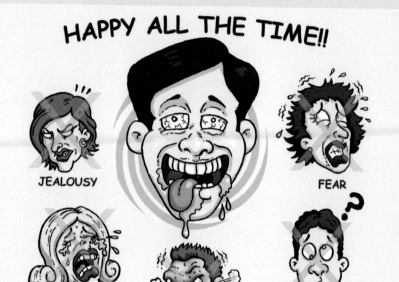

ARE YOUR EMOTIONS GETTING YOU DOWN?
LIFE IS TOO SHORT!
WHEN YOU CAN BE ...

HAPPY ALL THE TIME!!

JEALOUSY

FEAR

SADNESS

RAGE

CONFUSION

TRY OUR NEW ECSTALWAYS

SIDE EFFECTS INCLUDE FEELING ROMANTIC AT INAPPROPRIATE TIMES, A FUNKY ODOR, UNCONTROLLABLE GIGGLING, LIVER FAILURE AND SUDDEN DEATH. ASK YOUR DOCTOR IF ECSTALWAYS IS RIGHT FOR YOU.

CHAPTER 9

# EMOTIONS

*There can be no transforming of darkness into light and apathy into movement without emotion.*                    *~Carl Jung*

Have you ever met those people who seem to be happy all the time? No matter what the situation, they tend to find the good aspects and they don't hang on to anger very long.

Then there are other people who see the negative, no matter how good everything is. They can get mad, stay mad, and hold onto grudges for years.

We are emotional creatures. We feel happy, joyful, bored, angry, and depressed. Emotions play a role in our daily lives at every moment, sometimes very strong emotions. Emotions drive us to act and how we deal with our emotions can greatly affect our quality of life.

How do we learn to handle and process our emotions?


## DEFINITION

Emotions are defined as:

> *An affective state of consciousness in which joy, sorrow, fear, hate, or the like, is experienced, as distinguished from cognitive and volitional states of consciousness.*[119]

Emotions are, in essence, *energy in motion*. They are a normal part of our existence.

We have all felt the extreme of emotions. A strong emotional health is essential to one's total health and wellbeing. Everyone has felt joy and happiness, in addition to anger, hurt, pain, depression, or suffered a broken heart.

## STATISTICS

- Americans spent $11.6 billion on antidepressants in 2010.[120]

- Anxiety Disorders affect about 40 million Americans (about 18%) each given year.[121]

- In a list of top therapeutic classes of drugs sold on market, antidepressants were ranked second, with 253.6 million prescriptions filled.[122]

- More than a quarter of Americans taking antidepressants have never been diagnosed with any of the conditions the drugs are typically used to treat.[123]

## DEALING WITH EMOTIONS

Most of us have not been taught how to deal with emotions in a healthy way.

When growing up, many of us have heard:

"Stop crying, baby!"

"Aw, he's having a tantrum!"

"Don't be scared, chicken!"

As children, we learn how to deal with emotions from watching our parents. Some parents handle them well. They are able to feel them, express the feelings in healthy ways, and then let them go. Some stifle their emotions, often causing feelings to build up, and then they explode every so often. Some fathers never express any emotions.

Often times when we express our emotions we are mocked or belittled, so some learn to hide and smother their emotions. We often try not to feel emotions and hope they'll go away.

Many of us were never taught how to properly handle our emotions. Have you met those people that seem to be stuck in anger? No matter what happens, they respond with rage and stay angry at things that happened long ago while others have moved on and forgotten about it. How long should someone stay angry and when and how should they be able to let the feelings go? Is it hard to believe that hanging on to anger or sadness, or any negative emotion can eventually progress into physical health problems?

## MEDICATIONS FOR EMOTIONS

*If you have an undesirable emotion, you can mask it, squeeze it, suppress it, displace it, hide it, exaggerate it, or fake it. Or you can ask the doctor for advice, and he may recommend some medication. If you're depressed, you can get Prozac which will add some serotonin and make you feel better. If you're anxious, you can get Valium or Xanax to calm you down. If you feel too happy and then too sad, or if you're bipolar, there's lithium. If you're angry too often: maybe a coke and a smile.*

There are medications for emotions that earn the drug companies huge profits. Yet many antidepressants have severe side effects. Some even increase the risk of suicidal behavior in children and young adults.[124]

There are a plethora of anti-anxiety medications that calm people down temporarily. Often patients become dependent upon them to regulate their emotions. Yet the anti-anxiety medications are addictive, and therefore controlled substances. If there's ever a problem where the patient lose their medication or don't have access to it for some reason, there's even more anxiety.

**143**

Besides the severe side effects and the potential addictive effect, is it a good idea to take these drugs? Shouldn't emotions be handled without drugs? People taking the medications are learning to mask their emotions and are not given effective tools or techniques to handle their emotions in healthy, natural ways.

When do emotions become conditions to be treated and disease states rather than natural forms of expression? Pharmaceutical treatments used to be for extreme cases, now they are used all too often. Pills are an easy way out, a patch on a problem that's not only convenient but also covered on insurance.

How about sadness or depression? Prolonged illness, divorce, and death of a family member are all reasons to feel sad for certain periods of time. Grieving is normal and feeling sad is normal. But at what point does it become a condition to be treated rather than a normal experience of life?

Antidepressants and anti-anxiety medications are a $20 billion per year industry.[125]

Is there a better way to deal with emotions than drugs?

Yes.

## NOTHING IS AS IMPORTANT AS THE WAY YOU FEEL— ABRAHAM

In fact, emotions are like waves that come through you. They cannot, and should not, be avoided. They are meant to be felt, and expressed.

Abraham, a non-physical teacher, speaks through Esther Hicks who currently teaches workshops around the world. The main purpose is to help guide people to feel better about their situation, whether minor or major, from being cut off in traffic, to having been raped. Abraham Hicks states that emotions are part of your guidance system to help you make decisions throughout your life.

According to the teachings of Abraham, "nothing is as important as the way you feel." The first few times I heard that I glazed over it, but then one day I got it. You start listening to your body; listen to what makes you feel lighter and what give you a greater feeling of relief. You learn to avoid situations and thoughts that create tension or make you feel bad. Or you change the thoughts about a situation, and feel how your body responds.

## THOUGHTS LEAD TO EMOTIONS

Our thoughts about any situation lead to our emotions. Whatever we think about and however we interpret a situation can create our emotions. We have control of our thoughts. Yet our minds are cluttered with advertisements, bad stories from the news, gossip, and other unhealthy things that dominate in much of our modern society.

In every situation in life we can train our minds to think more useful and beneficial thoughts. We can look at situations and choose what meaning we want to give to them.

Example 1:  Road rage

A car veers into your lane causing you to use the brakes to avoid a collision.

*Thought: That person cut me off. That person must feel that his path is more important than my own. He has no consideration for my boundaries. I'm going to make him pay for that! Today is a bad day! He must think I'm not worthy. He's right, I'm not worthy.*

*New thought: That guy must be late for something. I'm glad I left early and I'm not rushing around stressing like a maniac. He's creating his own stress. His experience has nothing to do with my own except for the meaning I give it. Good luck, I hope you make it to your destination.*

Example 2:  Greetings

A neighbor walks by and doesn't acknowledge or greet you.

*Thought: He's a snob. He must think he's better than me and must be too good to greet a neighbor.*

*New thought: He must be busy. Many people don't greet people that they don't know; it doesn't have anything to do with me.*

These are important habits to create. According to Abraham, that is our work—to create thoughts to make us feel better and may give us some feelings of relief. Everything that happens can be interpreted in a way that is beneficial to us.

It is a practice and it takes time to make it a consistent habit, but it's well worth the time.

Our thoughts lead to our emotions, which determine which words we speak, which lead to action. Everything starts with our thoughts, which we in fact have control. Learning how to actively create the most empowering thoughts is a healthy step towards dealing with emotions.

## EMOTIONS AND DISEASE

Is it hard to believe that poor processing of emotions can lead to physical health conditions? Western medicine does not associated emotions with disease. Yet from a holistic perspective, emotions are the basis underlying every health condition, from depression to heart disease and diabetes.

## Louise Hays[126]

Author of *Heal Your Life*, which was first written in 1976, is one of the original contributors of the self-help movement. She shows the connection of the emotions and mind to physical ailments of the body. She explains how our beliefs and ideas about ourselves are often the cause of our emotional problems and physical conditions and how, by using certain tools, we can improve our thinking, our lives and our health.

**146**

## HEALTHY WAYS TO DEAL WITH EMOTIONS

Many people are not taught how to deal with emotions. Often people make great efforts to not feel painful emotions, including by using drugs and alcohol to dull the senses, or numb the pain.

What is the correct way to handle emotions? Here are some tools that one can use to handle emotions:

**Express them.** Do not try to suppress them with the next supposedly great drug on the market.

**Forgive.** Forgive everyone and everything for anything in the past. It is unhealthy to hold a grudge or to be bitter years after an incident. If you don't know how to forgive, then as a first step set an intention that you want to be able to forgive everyone.

**Forgive yourself.** This is an important step in the healing process.

**Breathe deep.** Get oxygen circulated throughout the body, which releases toxins, helps deal with emotions, relieves tension, brings clarity, and relaxes both the mind and body.

**Emotional Guidance Scale.** Created by Abraham, when you are feeling an emotion, identify where on the chart that emotion lies. Then allow yourself to feel that emotion as much as possible. In fact, invite the emotion in so you can feel it completely, and then let it go. Then modify your thoughts about the situation to find a feeling higher in the chart. It's about finding a thought that feels better and then working your way up the chart.

For example, if you are depressed about a situation, let yourself feel the sadness and depression, allow the feelings in completely. Then try and view that situation in a way that makes you feel an emotion higher on the scale, like anger. This is working up the emotional scale as anger is more empowering and feels better than depression and powerlessness. Then let yourself feel the anger. Slowly change the thoughts to keep moving up the scale. Notice when your body feels relief versus tension.

**147**

---

**Emotional Guidance Scale**

1. Joy/Appreciation/Empowered/ Freedom/Love
2. Passion
3. Enthusiasm/Eagerness/ Happiness
4. Positive Expectation/Belief
5. Optimism
6. Hopefulness
7. Contentment
8. Boredom
9. Pessimism
10. Frustration/Irritation/ Impatience
11. Overwhelment
12. Disappointment
13. Doubt
14. Worry
15. Blame
16. Discouragement
17. Anger
18. Revenge
19. Hatred/Rage
20. Jealousy
21. Insecurity/Guilt/Unworthiness
22. Fear/Grief/Depression/Despair/ Powerlessness

---

The Emotional Scale is created by Abraham-Hicks,
© by Jerry & Esther Hicks, Ask and it is Given,
AbrahamHicks.com
(830) 755-2299

**Release Emotions.** Find healthy ways to release intense emotions. Hitting a pillow, exercising, writing freehand, dancing, or even therapy are all ways to let go of emotions.

**Emotional Freedom Technique (EFT).**[127] EFT is a form of psychological acupressure, simple tapping with the fingertips while thinking about a problem. It is based on the same energy meridians used in traditional acupuncture, but without the needles. It has been used to treat physical and emotional ailments, including traumatic events, addictions, and pain. It has been in use for over five thousand years.

**Somatic Experiencing.**[128]  A technique that helps with accumulated stress, involves orienting oneself to pleasure and also creating an awareness of how emotions are felt in different areas of the body.

**12 Step Programs.**[129]  Like alcoholics anonymous and overeaters anonymous, the 12-step programs recognize that addictive behaviors have connections with past pain and guilt. One of the steps involves making amends to those you have wronged, and forgiving yourself and others.

**Be part of a Community.**  Being part of a community helps people belong and also serves as a support system.

## SUMMARY

Emotions are another aspect of our lives where the drug industry has learned how it can make huge profits. Yet many of the drugs serve as temporary solutions and often have terrible side effects. People can be taught healthy and natural ways to handle even the most intense emotions.

## POINTS TO REMEMBER:

- Experiencing a range of emotions is a normal part of our lives.

- Emotions should be felt completely, and then released.

- Drugs for emotions have some severe side effects, and patients are not taught how to deal with emotions in healthy and natural ways.

- There are many natural techniques to assist people in dealing with emotions.

## INTERVIEW WITH SOMATIC EXPERIENCING AND YOGA PRACTITIONER SONYA ARAGON

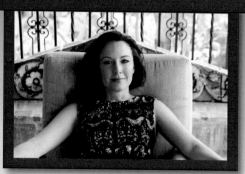

*Growing up, Sonya was at the top of her class, well-liked, and a trusted neighborhood babysitter. At 16, she developed an all-consuming addiction to stimulants. For a decade, she cycled through periods of high achievement and self-destruction. Sonya graduated college a year early, then taught and did research in Asia and Central America, and went to graduate school on a paid assistantship. After a series of car accidents and overdoses, destroying her budding career, and nearly losing her leg to an embolism, she underwent heart surgery at the age of 26.*

*Sonya resolved her addictive behavior and developed a healthy range of emotions through practices based on cultivating body awareness and orienting to pleasure. These practices include Somatic Experiencing, the Anat Baniel Method, and yoga. She now provides a supportive environment for children and adults to experience the here and now, resolve physical and psychological limitations, and relieve symptoms of trauma, stress, and chronic pain.*

**Dr. Leyla: What was your childhood like?**
Sonya: Born a preemie and incubator baby, I was the eldest of three kids, with my sister four years younger and my brother eight years younger. My father runs a small business and my mother is a nurse. I have a close-knit extended family, matriarchal and Catholic. A lot of my family members have trouble with anxiety, but they tend to use food to regulate their mood more than alcohol or other drugs.

**Dr. Leyla: Did you have problems as a child?**
Sonya: I always had digestive and anxiety problems, but I couldn't really name them because I had no other point of reference and I was so disconnected from my body. I was unhappy much of the time, and unable to experience simple pleasures.

**Dr. Leyla: How did you respond to this as a child?**
Sonya: I felt stressed all the time, like I was in a panic attack 24 hours per day. Except I didn't know it, because I didn't know you could feel differently. I was insecure, anxious, depressed, and yearning for connection. As I got older I discovered self-medicating and the thrill of high risk behaviors. It was the only time I could feel anything.

**Dr. Leyla: Did this affect your performance in school?**
Sonya: I did well in school, grade-wise. Although I didn't have the language or body awareness to identify my anxiety problems, my academic achievement was the lynchpin of my sense of survival and my only real means for being seen and validated.

**Dr. Leyla: Were you able to develop normal friendships and relationships?**
Sonya: I was extremely socially delayed. I had few templates for two-way, caring communication. I couldn't feel myself, so I really couldn't feel other people. I tried to turn every available adult into a parent figure. I also took refuge in creating a persona, but I only succeeded in alienating people further.

**Dr. Leyla: When you got older were you able to get help for your health problems and anxiety?**
Sonya: The first intervention I received was pharmaceutical, and ineffective. I also received conventional talk therapy off and on. It helped some, but it often exacerbated my physical symptoms and subsequent behaviors. It wasn't until I discovered Somatic Experiencing after my heart surgery that I experienced lasting change and relief.

**Dr. Leyla: As a teenager, what was your life like? Did the anxiety and stomach problems continue?**
Sonya: I didn't have the language or the tools to deal with emotional or anxiety problems. So instead I leaned on drugs. I had this really creative year when I was 15 that involved painting and sewing. As soon as I started driving, though, I started using drugs, namely crystal methamphetamine and marijuana.

**Dr. Leyla: Did you get into trouble?**
Sonya: I crashed a car and fought with my parents frequently, but no one knew I was using until I ran away from home at 16.

**Dr. Leyla: How long were you gone and why did you come back?**
Sonya: I was gone for just over a week, and was taken in by a kind professional juggler who was filling his apartment with lost souls off the Venice boardwalk. The police picked me up in my car for a minor traffic infraction.

When I got back I was institutionalized for two weeks at a private hospital. I was incorrectly diagnosed with bipolar disorder on the basis of my responses to a questionnaire and forcibly medicated. I remember how childlike I felt in there. I was terrified, ashamed, and I longed for comforting human contact—to have my hand held or to be told I wasn't worthless. I still remember the two staff members who treated me with dignity. I had to really fight to continue seeing the therapist there I felt safe with and found helpful. The psychiatrist that ran the adolescent ward used a treatment approach that revolved around negating everything I felt and said. That kind of continual criticism had a lot to do with how I ended up there in the first place.

**Dr. Leyla: What happened when you got out?**
Sonya: When I went home I started therapy. It was helpful because it was the first time that I became aware that I had feelings inside my body that made me do things. Previously, everything was on impulse and I just took action, often in very damaging ways. I had no awareness of the internal sensations of emotions. When I worked through talk therapy, however, it would stir things up without allowing my physical stress responses to compete.

**Dr. Leyla: So it was helpful?**
Sonya: Yes, it was the first time that I had an adult who I could trust, a more neutral party to talk things out with. He validated my feeling that I needed some replacement for the parenting I received. I learned to allow myself to feel the emotions inside my body and to be present.

**Dr. Leyla: Did you finish high school?**
Sonya: Even though I almost dropped out a few times, I had a 4.0 grade point average until I started drinking and driving and using drugs. I was still able to go to a university. When I went to college, my therapist didn't mention that I might want to continue care. I felt a lot of shame for needing this kind of help, so I didn't continue any therapy.

**Dr. Leyla: Where did you go to college?**
Sonya: Right after I finished high school I got certified in massage therapy. Then I went to UC Santa Cruz.

**Dr. Leyla: How were your college years? Did you continue using drugs?**
Sonya: I tapered off pot smoking in the first year, and by the second year I was using methamphetamine intermittently. I really liked the feelings from it because it was self-medicating—it got rid of my depression and anxiety, and it made me feel powerful, energized, and creative. I was also a binge drinker.

**Dr. Leyla: But you still made it through school?**
Sonya: I was able to graduate early with a degree in biology. I had a bit of course credit already accumulated when I entered college from taking the advanced placement tests in high school.

**Dr. Leyla: And then what happened after college?**
Sonya: While working as a massage therapist and waiting for an internship placement in Southeast Asia, I got a DUI and shattered my leg. I had hardware put into my leg. Then I had a botched wisdom tooth extraction that exposed the nerve of another tooth. Hoping to avoid a lawsuit, the dentist prescribed me Vicodin. These back-to-back experiences gave me a taste for opiates. I eventually recovered and worked in Singapore for a month at the botanic gardens. Then I went to Northeast Thailand for a year where I taught and helped a professor write a book on medicinal plants.

**Dr. Leyla: Then did you finally get help?**
Sonya: No. When I was applying to graduate schools, I started using cocaine pretty heavily. It lasted for about a year.

**Dr. Leyla: Was this your rock bottom?**

Sonya: No. I went to grad school. After a semester, I started injecting morphine. And then I started adding cocaine to my morphine. After a night of binging, I was teaching a biology lab when I fell asleep standing up in front of the class. This happened during the last semester of my master's degree. Consequently, I wasn't able to finish.

**Dr. Leyla: Was that your rock bottom?**

Sonya: No. At this point, I became a full time user. I was addicted to opiates, and I was also injecting cocaine every day. I wasted away to 93 pounds and developed a 103°F fever that I let go for a month. I was a few days away from dying of heart failure, lying in the back seat on our way to our dealer's house when my friend fell asleep at the wheel and rolled our car. My boyfriend slammed into my chest and dislodged some blood clots which caused two embolisms—one in my spleen and one in my leg. I waited a day before going to the hospital.

**Dr. Leyla: What happened at the hospital?**

Sonya: I remember seeing the horrified looks on their faces—my leg was cold and white and I was very close to needing to have it amputated. They couldn't get me into the operating room fast enough. I also had a severe heart infection, endocarditis, from introducing skin bacteria into my blood stream. I was only a few days away from heart failure and at 26 years old I had open heart surgery, specifically mitral valve replacement.

**Dr. Leyla: Was this your rock bottom?**

Sonya: Yes, although I really don't remember much of the next two weeks. They had me heavily sedated. My mom was waiting by my hospital bed when I woke up. I went back home to California and then to rehab.

**Dr. Leyla: How was rehab?**

Sonya: I detoxed in rehab, but I also relapsed a couple of times. It was there that I learned about a retreat center. So I went to stay in the desert and do yoga.

**Dr. Leyla: How did you learn to deal with the addictions and other issues?**
Sonya: I started working with Somatic Experiencing four years ago. My body learned, for the first time, how to land in a relaxed, but alert state after becoming distressed at that primitive, brain stem level. I had no capacity to self-soothe prior to this.

**Dr. Leyla: Is that when you discovered the holistic world?**
Sonya: I had been oriented toward traditional medicine and natural healing since high school, but this was the first time I was learning a model that was urgently relevant to my own life, that incorporated what I learned studying evolutionary biology, and supported my yoga practice. I was able to start learning how to let my emotions move through me instead of take me over. Before this I was disconnected, impulsive, and lonely. Now I walk around with a sense of pleasure and well-being I never knew before. My social skills are also getting better. A big part of that comes from living in a community of yoga practitioners. It gets easier and easier for me to connect to other human beings.

**Dr. Leyla: How does Somatic Experiencing work?**
Sonya: It is a method for the release of trauma, or accumulated stress from the nervous system. It helps one move from being overwhelmed and disoriented to orientation and ease. It works with the whole brain—the neocortex, limbic brain, and the brain stem to develop a sense of one's associations and complete self-protective responses to bring the nervous system back to a relaxed, yet alert state.

**Dr. Leyla: What do you mean by "accumulated stress"?**
Sonya: Trauma is defined by response to stimuli, not any external measure of the severity of an event. Different individuals have varying levels of resilience, or ability to restore balance when stressed. We live in a novel, manufactured world hallmarked by overstimulation and disconnection. When adrenaline kicks in, we are in the fight or flight response. This is our body's response to danger and is a survival mechanism. It is only meant to be like that for a few moments at a time.

However, modern people are exposed to a multitude of stressors without much time or means for deactivation in between. We may spend a lot of time in that fight or flight response, which our bodies are not created for. In time, this stress accumulates and leads to a state of *freeze* marked by numbness, lack of expression, and low energy. Chronic freeze and chronic fight-or-flight have their own sets of health problems, and people who bounce between those two states are often misdiagnosed as having bipolar disorder.

**Dr. Leyla: Why are so many people overloaded with stress?**
Sonya: It's a social epidemic. We are walking around with a hunter gatherer nervous systems in an alien environment. The world is changing at a much faster rate than our bodies have adapted. We are intensely social creatures, designed to function in small cooperative groups where everybody knows each other. It's increasingly challenging for people to bond that closely even to one's own children these days. That trend is truly ominous. Experiencing strong caretaking bonds in the early years lays the foundation for resilience in the face of stress. What happens to our society as a whole if fewer and fewer individuals are equipped to fully engage with each other and face life's challenges?

**Dr. Leyla: Can you describe a session of Somatic Experiencing?**
Sonya: For a talk-based, seated session, we start by noticing the room to orient and find things we like to look at or listen to or smell. Then we allow our attention to move inward to something pleasant. The tough stuff comes on its own. When it does, we notice it, describe it a bit, and move back to experiences that are comforting or pleasurable. We are also looking for behaviors—movements that may be supportive or self-protective.

**Dr. Leyla: Would you describe emotions as "Energy in Motion"?**
Sonya: I think that's an accurate description and a powerful reminder. For me, that translates to locating the sensation of emotion in my body, and then watching how that changes. It helps remind me that the emotions will flow, change, and pass through. Is there heat? Are my legs shaking? Where in my body am I experiencing the emotion? This general process is common to many contemplative traditions. The powerful

thing about Somatic Experiencing is that it incorporates an understanding of the physiological mechanisms that drive this process and which we share with trauma-free wild animals.

**Dr. Leyla: But if you are not expressing the emotions, aren't you suppressing them?**
Sonya: No, you can express them, but if you sit with them and observe them, it is actually more powerful than acting them out. In this model, when we do act on self-protective motor impulses, we do it very slowly for its completion to register in the cerebellum. You can also offset the emotions by orienting to pleasure, focusing your attention elsewhere, or imagining it's opposite. Emotions are always changing, although it doesn't always feel so in more traumatized, stuck nervous systems. Even with a panic attack there is a rush of adrenaline, but it only acts in the body for 10 minutes at a time, which can, of course, feel more like an hour.

**Dr. Leyla: People often have unresolved childhood traumas that they hold with them. Does one have to relive bad experiences, for example, scream at their parents, or their abuser, in order to resolve these issues?**
Sonya: Quite the opposite. Violence begets violence via the large proportion of mirror neurons in the motor cortex. Most of my clients have developmental trauma that manifests in their adult life as anxiety, chronic pain, addiction, or intimacy issues. You deactivate the emotional charge around experiences surrounding an event by orienting to pleasure and attending to sensation or image. You can separate out different parts of your experiences. If you attend to your nervous system, you expand your capacity. Then you have more compassion for the way the big people were; it's easier to understand their personal pain, limitations and lack of awareness.

**Dr. Leyla: They say we should forgive everyone and everything— does Somatic Experiencing help you do that?**
Sonya: It does in that it helps you understand the three phases of the nervous system we're all working with—social engagement and orientation, fight or flight, and freeze. If you can discern which phase is dominant for someone, it's easier to sense what it feels like where they're coming from.

**Dr. Leyla: How should people be taught to deal with emotions?**
Sonya: Orienting to pleasure is a good place to start, even if that means focusing on something neutral. It helps to keep in mind that emotions are a form of currency that evolved in social animals to help keep track of which relationships are beneficial for survival. It is helpful to learn how to tolerate strong sensations. Then you can recognize the emotion, track the sensations, images, and thoughts associated with it; and reorient to what or who is pleasant, beautiful, and comforting around you.

**Dr. Leyla: They say that people often learn to deal with their emotions through their parents. How did your parents deal with their emotions?**
Sonya: My parents were very dedicated to their children. They did their best to give us all we needed. However, love is learned. My parents didn't have much experience with being emotionally available, physically affectionate, or attuned to reading or allowing for our feelings.

**Dr. Leyla: As a former addict, do you ever struggle with cravings to alcohol or drugs?**
Sonya: Rarely, if ever. I am getting better at observing and containing my emotions all the time. I recently took a narcotic following a minor medical procedure and now I find the mood-altering effects more annoying than entertaining. My body feels better without drugs or alcohol than it does with it. I went from having a stuck, all-or-nothing nervous system to experiencing more moderate ups and downs, situationally appropriate responses, and a general sense of pleasure in being alive.

**Dr. Leyla: Can Somatic Experiencing help those who struggle with addictions?**
Sonya: Yes. This method addresses the physiological dysregulation that motivates addictive behavior in the first place. It conditions the body to provide its own relief, which is both more immediate and more reliable than any external source could provide. We are exquisitely sensitive social creatures. The soothing we get from our habits we can relearn how to get from each other. Being with animals and natural landscapes can also bring us to that relaxed, aware state.

**Dr. Leyla: What is your life like today?**
Sonya: I joke that I'm semi-retired, and there's a grain of truth to it. I used to be go-go-go. I felt like I had to constantly perform and achieve just to earn the right to be alive. I've gradually shifted from doing to being. I enjoy spending time with my husband, my extended family and the other yoga practitioners in my community. I don't derive my sense of self-worth from my accomplishments any longer. I love just exploring the world as I am.

**Dr. Leyla: How do you want to help others?**
Sonya: I want to communicate to as many people as possible that social engagement, relating to one another, is a part and parcel of having a physically healthy nervous system. With trauma resolution, functional movement, and yoga, I have something to offer everybody. Many of my clients come to me for pain, anxiety, and anti-aging. I'm working more and more with children. I help them deal with emotions through play. Left to their own devices, kids will reenact traumatic experiences without bringing them to resolution. Intervention can be as straightforward as helping them create happy endings. I practice the Anat Baniel Method for learning through movement, which produces remarkable outcomes for special needs kids.

I am also focused on expanding outside the narrow constraints of hour-slot healing appointments to provide my clients with a sense of community. I am hosting personal retreats for my clients at our yoga retreat center, and several clients have taken on daily practices in addition to office visits. Blending the therapeutic treatment model with the tradition of daily practice creates an abundance of opportunities for the nervous system to learn orientation and social engagement, the keys to landing the nervous system in a state of relaxed awareness.

**Sonya Aragon**
**(619) 233-3302**
**Sonya@webewell.org**

**WeBeWell.Org**

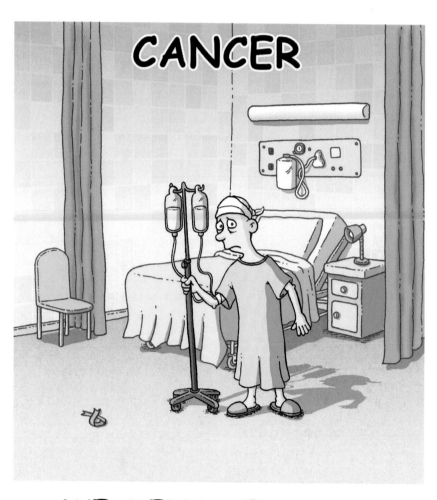

CHAPTER *10*

# CANCER

*We have a multi-billion dollar industry that is killing people, right
and left, just for financial gain. Their idea of research is to see whether
two doses of this poison is better than three doses of that poison.*
~Dr. Glenn Warner M.D.

A good friend of mine started getting pains in her stomach. She was
very conscious of her health and was active with no previous health issues.
She primarily ate a vegetarian diet, drank an abundance of green health
drinks, and was very aware of how thoughts affect one's health. She didn't
believe that cancer was a possibility for her because she was very educated
and in tune with the holistic lifestyle and cancer therapies. However, she
was diagnosed with ovarian cancer that had spread to her stomach. She
had a failed digestive tract and two colostomy bags. After trying different
therapies, including chemotherapy and ozone therapy in Mexico, she
passed away at the young age of 35.

I was at the Optimum Health Institute in San Diego when I first met Bill.
At 63 years old, he could barely eat, and was struggling to move. Bill was
in bad shape. He had prostate cancer that had spread to his bones. The
doctors had given him a few months to live and some strong medications
to make him more comfortable for his final months.

The Optimum Health Institute provided a cleansing and detoxification
diet, unlimited access to the wheat grass room, as well as classes to teach
about the body, mind and spirit. By the end of the week, Bill was eating
two plates of food and walking with a fresh energy. That was over a year
ago and he continues to do well.

## CANCER STATISTICS

More and more people are getting cancer at younger ages. Cancer is the second leading cause of death after heart disease. Four in ten people will experience some type of cancer. One in three women will get breast cancer.[130]

## CANCER

Why are so many people getting cancer? Why does one patient survive and another dies?

If you're like most of the American population, you know someone that has experienced cancer or possibly you've had to deal with a cancer diagnosis yourself. For many people, cancer has somehow touched their lives.

There is a lot of fear associated with getting that cancer diagnosis. There is a fear of death, and also knowing that the western medicine's response to cancer treatment is difficult, toxic, and often can cause long-term and debilitating side effects. The standard treatment options offered by the medical doctor include radiation, chemotherapy, or surgery. After diagnosis, there is a long and difficult journey to go through before the cancer goes into remission, that is, if the patient survives both the cancer and treatment.

Cancer treatment is one of the best examples of how far off-course and disturbing western medicine has come in creating profit out of disease, all at the expense of the patient's health and wellness.

We live in a world where we can clone sheep, video chat with someone on the other side of the planet, send people to the moon, and carry thousands of songs in a device smaller than the palm of our hand. In the medical field there has been amazing progress, such as simple surgeries to correct the vision, organ transplants that save lives and prosthetic legs that can enable an amputee to run a marathon.

*Yet with cancer treatment, how can it be that the best solution our cutting-edge medical field has to offer is to load the patient with chemicals and practically*

**162**

*kill them as routine procedure to beat the cancer?*

## WESTERN MEDICINE CANCER TREATMENT

The only treatments that western medicine doctors are trained in are chemotherapy, radiation, and surgery. Legally doctors can only recommend these treatments to their patients. These are also the only treatments that doctors can legally recommend to their patients.[131]

**Chemotherapy**[132] works by giving the patient powerful chemical drugs which kills the fast growing cancer cells. It also slows the growth of cancer cells and keeps the cancer from spreading in the body. It kills other fast growing cells in the body as well, such as cells of the stomach and intestines, hair follicles, and bone marrow cells that produce blood cells.

Side effects can include nausea and vomiting, hair loss and low blood cell count. Low red blood cells can lead to anemia. Infections are more likely to occur when there is a low white cell count. And low platelet counts can cause easy bleeding and bruising.

**Radiation therapy**[133] uses high doses of radiation to kill cancer cells. Low dose radiation is used for x-rays. Radiation for cancer works the same way, but with higher doses.

**Surgery** cuts the cancer out of the body.

## PROBLEMS WITH CANCER TREATMENT

### Doctor Training

Although most believe that medical doctors are trained to offer the best solutions for our health, the profession has evolved into one that is trained in the profitable therapies only. Cancer treatments, consisting of surgery, chemotherapy, and radiation have become accepted as the standard cancer treatment protocols, but not because they are the most effective—only because they are the most profitable. Yet these are the only therapies that medical doctors typically learn in their standard education.

**163**

## Chemotherapy and Radiation

Many may argue that chemotherapy and radiation work. But the question is: at what cost? A common analogy is burning down your house to get rid of termites. The termites may be gone, but the house structure is severely damaged if not destroyed. Similarly, chemotherapy and radiation may work, but after adding toxic chemicals to your body, the patient can experience a host of debilitating side effects for years to come.

## Suppression of Holistic Therapies

Although we often hear people within the mainstream media speak of "finding a cure" for cancer. Actually, there are cures that the Federal Drug Administration (FDA) and the American Medical Association (AMA) have fought against, all in the name of profit. It's hard to believe that our country is so wrong when it comes to cancer treatment. As discussed in Chapter 2, there have been non-toxic and successful cancer treatments in the past that were actually suppressed by the AMA and FDA.

To review the history of the suppression of cancer treatments, there are two incidents that stand out (previously mentioned in Chapter 2):

- Royal Rife built a *Rife Machine* in the 1930s after discovering that certain frequencies kill microorganisms, without harming the healthy cells. Despite the fact that it worked, his equipment was confiscated and his laboratories were destroyed. Some of the doctors were harassed to the point of quitting the profession. Rife was basically bullied and put out of business.[134,135]

- Secondly, in the 1940s there was the Hoxsey Treatment which consists of a caustic herbal paste for external cancers or an herbal mixture for internal cancers, combined with laxatives, douches, vitamin supplements, and dietary changes. Despite the fact that he had cured hundreds of patients of cancer, the AMA and FDA launched a vicious attack against him and called his salve worthless and dangerous. In the 1960s his 17 clinics were closed by the FDA. Hoxsey treatment is now available in Tijuana, Mexico.[136]

**164**

## Cancer Laws

- Medical doctors are only allowed to prescribe chemotherapy, radiation and surgery for cancer treatment. Doctors can get disciplinary action or have the medical license revoked when using alternative or holistic therapies.[137]

- It is illegal to claim to *cure cancer*. The FDA or AMA will often use that as a reason to raid and close down clinics that offer natural and alternative treatments.[138]

- There are now reports of lawsuits where a child was diagnosed with cancer and the law required the child be treated with chemotherapy. Even though the side effects are severe and permanently damaging, and even though the parents choose to be treated with holistic alternatives, the courts ruled that it was illegal and their child must endure chemotherapy treatment.[139]

Medical doctor Michael Gerber was accused of inappropriately treating a potentially curable uterine cancer patient. He treated the patient for 27 months with a variety of holistic therapies including Hoxsey herbs, megavitamins, chelation therapy, Chaparral tea, pangymic acid, wheat grass, coffee or enzyme enemas, apricot pits, clover, and slippery elm.

Dr. Gerber claimed to have provided supplemental treatment to a patient who refused conventional treatment. Nevertheless, he was found guilty and his license to practice medicine in California was revoked in 1984 for gross negligence and incompetence, even though he had an otherwise clean record. The problem was in part due to the fact that he was using substances that had not been approved by federal or state authorities for the treatment of cancer.[140]

Is there logic to all this? How could natural treatments be so bad that it warrants arrest? Could anything be worse than chemotherapy, which works by killing fast-acting cancer cells AS WELL AS fast-acting healthy cells including bone marrow cells, digestive tract cells, and hair follicles? Chemotherapy is toxic. Yet it is the standard and accepted way to treat cancer in our society. It is approved by the government and medical profession.

**165**

## CANCER DEFINED

How you define and view cancer depends upon which school of thought you are coming from.

### Western Medicine Perspective

From the perspective of doctors and drugs, cancer consists of a large group of diseases, characterized by abnormal growth of cells, with these abnormal cells capable of migrating to other parts of the body.[141]

### Holistic Perspective

Everyone has cancer cells. If the body is healthy and balanced and the immune system is strong, the body can keep those cells in check and they will not become cancerous/malignant. Cancer takes a long time to develop as it takes time for a body to become out of balance, and there are several warning signs that may not have been noticed, or were simply ignored.

Cancer progression:

1. irritation
2. inflammation
3. lesion
4. induration (hardening) or tumor
5. cancer (malignancy)

## TREATMENT

### Western Medicine Perspective

When one is diagnosed with cancer by a medical doctor, it is a life changing moment. There is a certain feeling to it that is vulnerable, sick, helpless, and very fearful in the hands of the doctor who will make things better with radiation and chemotherapy. Patients must depend upon and listen to their doctor for greatest results. Causes of cancer can be hereditary, environmental, or otherwise random attacks on individuals. Treatments are

**166**

toxic and will create cancer-free or *fixed* patients with cancer in remission, yet they will be sicker in the long-term, and always fearful of a recurrence.

Western medicine does not take into consideration thoughts, emotions, or nutrition. It follows the pattern of creating long term customers that must rely on the expertise of doctors and drugs.

Western medicine treatment of cancer is very limited: Chemotherapy, radiation, and surgery to cut out the cancer.

## Holistic Perspective

With alternative medicine, the patient must discover what is creating the imbalance and take steps to learn about and heal him or herself. Patients must play an active role in their healing process. They must become empowered to learn what they need to do to heal themselves. Body, mind and spirit are all equally important and take into consideration nutrition, emotions, thoughts, and forgiveness. The healing process for cancer will boost the immune system, cleanse out toxins, and make the patient stronger, rather than harm the patient as in western medicine. The cancer takes a long time to develop, and the patient's health can gently be brought back to balance.

Cancer is viewed as a *Health Opportunity*, as one must stop their daily routine and pay attention to whatever is calling out to them. What do I need to learn? Who do I need to forgive? Healthy and empowering thoughts are used to regain balance. Thoughts include those of healing, visualizations of a healthy body, and of cancer being released. It is a time to release negative emotions.

Nutritionally, cancer is often caused by nutritional deficiencies and an imbalanced diet, which can create an acidic environment that is optimal for cancer to grow. Changing one's diet can quickly change the body from acid to alkaline and thus strengthen the immune system and heal the body. Additional steps to take include avoiding sugar as well as milk, since both feed cancer cell growth.[142]

Treatments are dependent upon the cause in each individual; they involve the examination of one's health including mind, body and spirit. The treatment consists of regaining balance, or going back to basics. Listen to your body. What is it trying to tell you? Cancer will force the patient to evolve into a being that has an awareness of the body, mind and spirit and is willing to let go of whatever is keeping them ill.

Going back to my friend that I mentioned earlier who passed at 35 years old, at the time I felt that cancer was a random attack on her as I knew she was vegetarian and very spiritual. However, after she found out that the man who she considered to be her soul mate was cheating on her, she didn't feel or express these emotions. She constantly dwelled upon it, as anyone would, yet she only tried to analyze why it happened. After learning more about cancer, I realized that she didn't deal with her troubling and heart breaking situation in a healthy or releasing way. Although she made the intention to do the right thing, part of being healthy is going through the emotions of the pain, allowing oneself to feel the hopelessness, sadness, anger, and rage, let oneself feel them completely, then let them go. She became numb to her emotions.

## NATURAL WAYS TO CURE CANCER

There are lots of ways to cure cancer, but don't expect your doctor to be knowledgeable about them. You must do your own research and often other countries have more options that are not available in the United States. Also remember that places within the United States cannot claim to *cure cancer*.

There are many alternative medicines cures or therapies for cancer, and the main goal is to regain the body's balance. What will work will depend upon what is causing the imbalance in the first place. The best approach for a patient is to attempt to regain balance in as many areas as possible. In essence, the journey of healing oneself of cancer will involve the body, mind, and spirit and will require that the patient evolve into a more open, self-aware, forgiving, self-empowered soul.

A mistake that many patients may make is to try one type of holistic therapy. Often the patient doesn't have any support from doctors or family, and once it doesn't work then they'll quickly jump back to western medicine's regimen of chemotherapy and surgery. However, it's necessary to jump in with both feet as there may be several issues that are off balance that need to be addressed. To heal oneself, a patient must first know and believe that it is possible to heal and the power lies within each person. They also must decide that they will make health a priority and do whatever is necessary to heal. It is necessary to address the issues on all levels, including mind, body and spirit, and do anything and everything possible to make the cancer disappear. If a person with cancer is already eating a vegetarian or vegan diet, then the cause may be emotional, etc.

Healing options include:

**Cleanse.** Get rid of the toxins, by cleansing, colonics, wheat grass, or choose from the many other techniques to cleanse toxins from the body.

**Raw Food.** Eliminate processed foods and sugars to help eliminate cancer. Processed foods add extra toxins to the body whereas the sugars create a more acidic environment that is favorable for cancer to grow. By eliminating these foods and eating only a raw food diet you are altering the environment to create a place where cancer cannot grow.

**Good Nutrition.** Eating raw food and other foods that are rich in nutrients and antioxidants will provide excellent source of vitamins and minerals and will help make the immune system stronger. It is important to provide enough nutrients so the body is strong, nourished, balanced and able to fight off diseases.

**Deal with Emotions.** Learning to deal with and express emotions in a healthy manner is important to regaining balance. Louise Hays teaches that forgiveness of everyone and for everything is important in releasing and regaining balance. Holding on to resentments can also lead to cancer.[143]

**Visualization/Hypnosis.** These two different techniques both encompass the power of the mind. The mind has amazing healing power that most do not know about or understand how to use. With visualization you learn to imagine the state of health that you wish to create. In hypnosis, you instruct your cells to be happy and healthy and give commands to your subconscious mind.

**Biomagnetism.** This technique works by adjusting the pH level in different areas of the body to restore balance. By adjusting the pH level to the normal and healthy range, the cancer cannot grow.

**Rife Machine.** Dr. Royal Rife, a microbiologist, designed his device to use different sound frequencies to kill microbes which were inside of the cancer cells without damaging the healthy cell. Then the cancer cells will be able to restore their metabolism and will revert into normal cells. It uses different sound frequencies based on the type of cancer cell. Originally created in the 1930s, with much success, the Rife Machine was suppressed by the FDA and AMA. It came back in the mid-1980s and is now available once again in the United States.[144]

**Ozone therapy.** Cancer cells cannot live in oxygen. Ozone therapy works by removing some of the blood, adding ozone which becomes oxygen, and then putting this oxygen-rich blood back into the body. Ozone therapy is not available in the United States. It is available in Germany and Mexico among other countries.[145,146]

**Vitamin C.** Linus Pauling studied the effects of vitamin C in the 1970s in treating cancer and found that his treatments increased the survival rate by four times.[147]

**Laetrile.** Laetrile is found in apple seeds, apricot seeds, and other seeds, and it has been used as a treatment for cancer since 1000 AD. Although it was discredited by the FDA in 1980, it has cured many people throughout the years.[148]

**Hoxsey Treatement.** Harry Hoxsey was the son of a veterinary doctor, although he was not a doctor. He used the formula created by his grandfather, which was originally used by the Native Americans. The Hoxsey treatment consists of two herbal formulas. One is external, and it consists of a red paste made with bloodroot, the active anti-tumor ingredient, mixed with zinc chloride and antimony sulfide. This paste is applied directly onto skin cancer tumors. The second is an herbal for internal cancers. Originally suppressed by the American Medical Association (AMA) and the Food and Drug Administration (FDA), the Hoxsey method can be found in Tijuana, Mexico.[149]

**170**

**Cancer Control Society.** This non-profit organization provides a great resource with information on alternative therapies and nutrition for cancer. www.CancerControlSociety.com

## SUMMARY

*It was actually very hard for me to believe that our government and entire health care system has gone so far astray that the best choices to treat cancer are suppressed and the more toxic though profitable therapies have become the standard. But that is the reality.*

There are many ways to cure cancer, just not in the United States. Generally, there is something wrong when the only approved methods are chemotherapy, drugs, radiation and surgery. The patient is exposed to toxins, left with a weakened immune system, and generally set up to take a downward spiral in their health.

Doctors are not trained in the best forms of healthcare, only the profitable ones that are endorsed by the pharmaceutical companies.

Contrary to what is taught in medical school, cancer is not a random invader that must be treated by giving your body over to the *experts*, rather it's a condition created when the body, mind and spirit is off balance and the problem is not addressed. Toxins in the body, unexpressed emotions, anger and resentment are all contributors to cancer and should be addressed.

In our culture, the belief system behind the cancer is one of the most damaging aspects. The patient is trained to feel like a helpless victim with statistical chances of recovering. The surgery will cut out a tumor, and then there will be radiation and chemotherapy that will practically kill the patient before they get better. In this case, listening to your doctor may be the worst thing that you can do for your body.

In the holistic world, cancer is easy to treat, and completely within the power of the individual. Rather than viewing the diagnosis as a horrible thing with a grim future, patients must gently discover which part of their life is off balance, and work to create optimal health in all areas of their lives. According to Abraham, "There is no physical body, no matter what the conditions, that cannot achieve an improved condition."[150]  Holistic treatments will not expose the patients to toxins; rather they will energize the body, empower the immune system, release negative emotions, and clear out the toxins. The patient must be empowered to know that the cure is within him or herself.

If diagnosed with cancer, do not rely on the expertise of a medical doctor for your entire treatment as there are many aspects to treatment and health that they are simply not trained in.


**POINTS TO REMEMBER:**

- United States doctors are only trained in chemotherapy, radiation, and surgery.

- There are many ways to heal cancer.

- Natural ways to cure cancer have been suppressed by the American Medical Association and the Food and Drug Administration.

- Healing cancer naturally involves the body, mind and spirit.

## INTERVIEW WITH CANCER SURVIVOR SUSAN MOSS

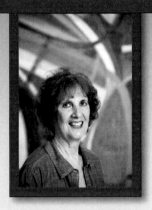

*Susan Moss was diagnosed with breast and uterine cancer after a devastating break up. Despite the insistence of her doctor, she refused surgery and chemotherapy. Instead she treated herself using natural and holistic methods. As the author of two books, **Keep Your Breasts** and **Survive Cancer**, Susan hopes to spread the message that you don't need surgery and toxic chemotherapy to treat cancer; you can heal yourself.*

**Dr. Leyla: What was your life like before?**
Susan: I had always been athletic. I kept myself fit by swimming and skiing. I was a girl scout, and then a lifeguard, and later on I taught skiing. I was also active in hiking, camping, and horseback riding. Although as an artist I was often under some financial stress.

**Dr. Leyla: What happened when you were diagnosed?**
Susan: The doctor found two tumors, one in the breast and the other in the uterus. The cancer showed up in the places in my body that had the most tension.

**Dr. Leyla: Why do you think you got cancer?**
Susan: I learned that the man of my dreams, who I thought was going to marry me, had actually married someone else. I was devastated and I really stopped taking care of myself for a year and a half after. I would still go to the gym but I would sit in the Jacuzzi and feel sorry for myself as I was extremely depressed and felt empty inside.

**Dr. Leyla: What did the doctor recommend?**
Susan: He insisted on surgery. When I told him that I refused, he was really upset. He actually called me every day, screaming at me and demanding I get the surgery.

**Dr. Leyla: Many people trust and believe their doctors as their health expert, and your doctor is calling you every day insisting that you follow his advice. How were you so certain that surgery and chemotherapy weren't for you?**

Susan: Two reasons. I had a close friend who was diagnosed with breast cancer, and I saw what they did to her—chemotherapy, radiation, mastectomy, and bone marrow transplant. She didn't ask any questions until soon before she died. She was a close friend; she was beautiful and only 38 years old when she passed. She died from the treatment, not the cancer. Secondly, in the seventies I healed myself from a tumor in my neck by using visualization techniques. So I knew it was possible. I also knew that if my friend would have let me guide her she would be here today.

**Dr. Leyla: How did you heal yourself of cancer?**

Susan: I did visualization techniques. While I was in the sauna I visualized the tumors melting away. When I was swimming I saw white light hitting my tumor and little white particles floating away. I visualized all day throughout the day. I decided to take my health back and regain control. I did a detox with whole grains, carrot juice, vegetable, fruits, minimal fish and no dairy so my body could clean out. I also took barley and wheat grass, both of which work like a vacuum to clean out toxins. I drank a lot of carrot juice, which is full of beta carotene. Studies have found that breast cancer patients are low in beta carotene. Spiritually I did a lot of praying and chanting. While I prayed and chanted I visualized what I wanted. It's magical what can happen when you can see the results. Visualizing yourself well and happy so you see the things you need is very powerful tool to get you to where you want to go. I also worked to get rid of anger and resentments. I did a lot through forgiveness and I learned to go on with my life. In addition, I did a lucky exercise where I would write down ten things that I'm lucky that I have, which is a form of gratitude exercise.

**Dr. Leyla: How long did it take you to heal yourself?**

Susan: It took me two months to get rid of the tumors, and seven more months to restore my health.

**Dr. Leyla: How did the doctor respond when you returned after healing yourself?**
Susan: When he couldn't find any tumors he was shocked. But after he was curious and asked me for information as he really wanted to know what I had done.

**Dr. Leyla: Why didn't you want the doctor to remove the tumors?**
Susan: Doctors will surgically remove the tumors, but actually the tumor is your friend.

**Dr. Leyla: What do you mean your *friend*?**
Susan: The tumor is trying to protect you; it's actually like an egg shell that holds the cancer cells, or like a dam that keeps water from flooding a city. Cutting into your body is the wrong thing to do when you are sick. Once your remove the tumor without treating the cause then the cancer spreads like wildfire. When you heal yourself and you don't have the tumor anymore, that is when you're healthy again.

**Dr. Leyla: Looking back, do you think you could have prevented your cancer?**
Susan: I was going through lots of emotional pain and depression for a year and a half. When you're grieving for whatever types of loss, you have to feel the pain and deal with the emotions. But I let myself go physically and emotionally. I think I could have prevented the cancer if I had dealt with the pain in more proactive healthy ways and maintained my exercise routine.

**Dr. Leyla: The statistics show that one in three women will get breast cancer, and four in ten will have some type of cancer. Why do you think so many people are getting cancer these days?**
Susan: There are high levels of stress and many people are emotionally distressed and lack the tools to deal with it. The medical community doesn't ask you anything about your life. This constant state of stress blocks the oxygen and hormones, and the high levels of adrenaline are what really cause the problems. Also nourishment is important as lots of people don't eat the proper things to be nourished, and our food is

depleted of minerals and vitamins. So many people aren't supplying their bodies with the nutrients needed to defend against a disease. There are also lots of pesticides and toxins in the home, like weed killers and cleaning products. People need to detox the mind, get rid of resentment, anger, and grudge holding. If there is anyone you're furious with, you must forgive them.

**Dr. Leyla: I understand that you created a program, MOTEP. Can you give some information on that?**
Susan: I originally created MOTEP to help heal myself. Soon after I was well I used the program to help others who were facing cancer. It stands for Marathon Olympic Tumor Eradication and Prevention program and it covers all the bases including spiritual, diet, exercise, emotions, laughing, chanting, prayer, visualization, etc. You must first decide you want to live and take control of your life. Secondly, you must decide that you will do anything it takes to get well. You must dedicate everything to your health. As part of this I also offered weekly group therapy for anyone with a problem mammogram to stage 4 cancers during which we talk about life, dance a little, do some creative activities, and some exercises to let go of anger, sadness or whatever problem emotion they are experiencing.

**Dr. Leyla: You wrote two books, *Keep Your Breasts* and *Survive Cancer*. Why did you write these?**
Susan: When I first went to the bookstore in 1988, I couldn't find a single book on preventing breast cancer. I wrote my first book in 1994, *Keep Your Breasts*, which is about my healing in contrast to my friend Kimberly, who did exactly what the doctor said and passed away at 38. She had everything going for her, so it was very tragic when she passed. Also she spent $350,000 for medical treatment, and I healed myself almost for free. I did pay to go to the gym, and for group therapy, yet I saved when I didn't buy meat or dairy. The costs were minimal in comparison.

**Dr. Leyla: And the second book?**
Susan: *Survive Cancer* is about people who used my program and were able to heal themselves, and also about individuals who figured out similar ways to heal themselves.

**Dr. Leyla: Do you have a program to maintain your health?**
Susan: Now I keep a diet high in vegetables, fruits, whole grains, nuts and seeds. I cut out all dairy except for yogurt. I work vigilantly to keep a healthy weight by working out, swimming, and lifting weights. I also strive to maintain a healthy and positive attitude.

**Dr. Leyla: What message would you want to tell people?**
Susan: When you heal yourself on every level you don't have recurrences—but you have to stay on that path and stay on the program the rest of your life. I now enjoy my life and my level of health very much.

**Susan Moss**
**4767 York Blvd.**
**Los Angeles, CA 90042**
**(323) 255-3382**

**SusanHMoss.com**
**SusanMossArt.com**

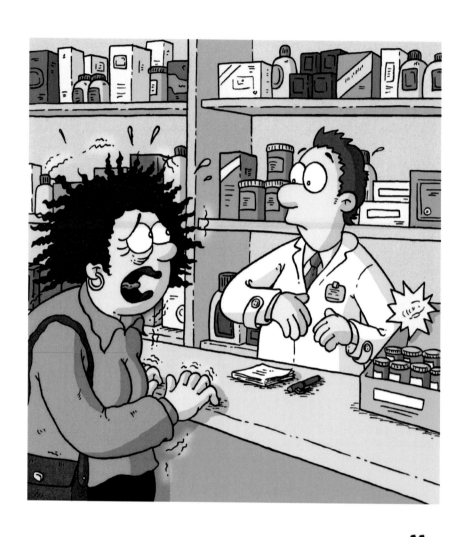

I NEED MY MEDICINE!!

## CHAPTER 11

# WHAT I HATE ABOUT PHARMACY

*The trouble with being in the rat-race is that even if you win, you're still a rat.*                    *~Lily Tomlin*

The intention of this chapter is to share a behind the scenes look at the struggles and difficulties in a pharmacist's daily work that many may not be aware of. Before pharmacy school I had a job in a pharmacy, so I knew what the daily life would be like. Yet it all felt different when I recieved my pharmacy license and landed there as final destination. It seemed false and misguided; there was little preparation for the *real world of pharmacy* in my school training. We were taught to expect that pharmacists were trusted and admired, but when in practice that is not always the case.

As a temporary, or relief pharmacist, I had the opportunity to experience work in a variety of pharmacy settings. My intention is to shed some light on the daily lives in your neighborhood pharmacy, with a touch of humor.

## CAGE LIFE

Working behind a cage all day—yes, this is a form of protection. There are lots of expensive and desirable drugs to protect. The truth is it often feels too much like a circus monkey on display.

## RUSH, RUSH

Everyone is in a hurry. Imagine for a moment being on the receiving end of a typical customer and their incessant questions—all day, every day:

"What's taking so long, you said twenty minutes?"

"I have food/ice cream/sick husband/dog in the car."

"Don't you just have to put some pills in a bottle?"

"Why is it not covered? I have insurance!"

"Where's the bathroom key?"

## ON MY FEET

Standing on my tired feet for eight or twelve hours a day takes a toll on the body. Where is my office with a view?

## FORGOT EVERYTHING

I forgot everything I learned in pharmacy school. We learned all kinds of things from anatomy, and biochemistry, to pharmacokinetics; or how a drug is absorbed, distributed throughout the body, and then eliminated. There's no use for this knowledge in retail pharmacy.

## TOO MANY BOSSES

Okay, so maybe I'm not totally a *people person*, but this is ridiculous, there are simply too many people to answer to; it's constant. Here are some of the folks that pharmacists must answer to:

**Corporate Clowns.** They are everywhere in today's world. In chain-store pharmacy, these bigwigs visit pharmacy locations unannounced in their fancy suits. They offer their puffed-up oversight skills by checking records for sales and profits, ensuring the store looks clean and presentable, making sure employees are wearing name tags and smiling, and pointing out any other problems that need attention.

**180**

**State Board of Pharmacy.** They conduct random checks to make sure the pharmacy is adhering to all federal and state pharmacy laws. Refrigerators must be at a certain temperature, pharmacists and technician licenses must be displayed, and rules and regulations must be followed.[151] These are the folks who have your pharmacy license in their hands. Don't get on their bad side!

**Store Manager.** At a large drug store the store manager handles the main store, and the pharmacy manager handles the pharmacy. I understand the importance of someone minding the shop while we dole out drugs, but some store managers can really overstep their boundaries in the pharmacy. There's often a potential for power struggle between the store manager and the pharmacy manager.

**Doctors.** I once questioned a doctor about the high dosage that he prescribed for a patient, since it was much higher than the manufacturer's recommended dose. I wondered if he had specialized in this area and wrote it intentionally, or did he simply make a mistake? I called to find out. His response:

"How much experiences have you had in prostate cancer? I've been studying this for 10 years."

Then he hung up the phone.

**Nurses.** They can be equally as difficult as doctors, and sometimes very stubborn. Here's a sample of a typical communication:

Pharmacist, "Can you please verify this dose with the doctor to make sure it's what he wanted?"

Uninterested in complying, the nurse responded, "No, it's right; it's what he wanted."

Pharmacist, "Can you double check with him please?"

The nurse persisted. "It's fine!"

**Pharmaceutical Representatives.** They come to the store locations

**181**

displaying glossy charts and graphs that promote the newest exciting drug on the market. In the past drug representatives would be the gift givers, armed with fancy pens, stuffed animals, and lunches for pharmacists and doctors. This was done in effort to educate, or promote really, the healthcare providers about their product to increase sales. The laws finally changed so that drug companies can no longer give these types of gifts, and their roles should be more educationally motivated.[152] Now pharmacists can listen to the product information for the drug without receiving gifts.

**Drug Enforcement Agency (DEA).** They are responsible for monitoring the controlled medications. These controlled medications are categorized by their potential for abuse and addiction. Products like oxycodone, morphine, and amphetamine are more controlled and therefore must be counted by hand on a monthly basis. Every single pill must be accounted for. Don't let this count be off!

**Health Insurance Auditors.** They have been on the prowl lately. The job of an insurance auditor is to come to the pharmacy and look through the stack of previously filled prescriptions to search for errors. If an error is found, or the pharmacy isn't following all insurance-provider policies, the insurance company doesn't have to pay the reimbursement for that prescription. I've witnessed an audit that included counting drops in an eye-drop prescription. They have also demanded reimbursement for medical supplies delivered to a nursing home when the patient had already passed away—even though the facility kept the supplies!

**Loss Prevention.** They monitor customers as well as employees to prevent theft. Another one who is watching us!

**Time clocks.** Yuck. Enough said.

## GOOD DAY / BAD DAY

A good day in many other careers, like sales, involves closing a deal, or signing a new account. Many industries reward their workers with incentives for exemplary effort—even paying a bonus above and beyond salary and benefits. In the pharmacy arena, bonuses are possible mostly for pharmacy managers, but not as common. A typical good day involves minimal interruptions or complaints from store customers, and a normal *bonus* is to have a day without the moans from a patient waiting too long for a prescription. A bad day is being overworked, understaffed, demanding and impatient customers, drug interactions, making a mistake, state board visit, dealing with phony prescriptions or addicts, and questions about constipation or diarrhea.

## THIEVES

As for the *risks* of pharmacy life, pharmacists hold the key to lots of desirable, addictive, and valuable drugs. Unfortunately, thieves and drug addicts know this. Thus, these drugs are kept enclosed, caged, and hopefully protected from robbery.

Here are some experiences with thieves, from my own personal interactions as well as those of coworkers:

1. In the past, insulin syringes were strictly monitored, and only available to those with diabetes. The drug addicts who simply wanted syringes would be creative in trying to obtain them. For example, a customer politely explained to me that he needed syringes so that his aunt could "shoot-up insulin." Also, there was an incident where, in an act of desperation, a person leaped over the counter to grab a box of syringes and then bolted from the store.

   Now the laws allow heroin addicts to buy a limited supply of syringes from certain pharmacies. Dirty needles can spread diseases such as HIV as well as Hepatitis C. Allowing addicts access to a clean supply of needles was determined to be the lesser of the two evils.

2. Once I was robbed at gunpoint for oxycontin. Since the street value is approximately $1 per milligram,[153] then one 80 milligram (mg) tablet might sell for $80, and a bottle with a hundred tablets could sell for $8,000! This high street value makes oxycontin a very desirable drug amongst thieves.

**183**

3. Phenergan with Codeine is a cough syrup and a favorite amongst a variety of thieves. The street value for a 16 ounce bottle is $300. A pharmacy technician threw full bottles in the trash, which were then recovered by her partner in crime out at the dumpster and sold for a nice profit. Apparently it makes a good cocktail when mixed with Sprite.

4. A pharmacy manager noticed that the Viagra inventory was constantly short. He started closely monitoring the automated ordering and the pill counts. He also had security install spy cameras and review the tapes. They found the janitors were pocketing the *little blue pill* as they swept the floors.

5. At my friend's store, during a busy rush, a woman walked through the employee entrance, dressed in the store's uniform and vest. This woman grabbed two bottles of Tussionex, a very strong cough syrup, placed them in a standard store tote, and proceeded to walk out. It was rush hour and there were several employees working in the pharmacy at the time. Although everyone else was preoccupied, my friend was the only one to notice the woman's actions and confronted her. The thief put up a huge fight like a wild animal, shattered one of the bottles, but at the end she was arrested.

6. A pharmacist stole a few hundred thousand dollars' worth of high priced drugs and sold to privately owned pharmacies for a nice discount. Security installed a spy camera and he was eventually caught.

7. A pharmacy technician ordered a special brand of amphetamine for her personal use. It wasn't a popular brand, so it went unnoticed for a long time. It was somewhat unfortunate when she finally got caught, since the drug made her a very speedy and efficient worker.

## FAKE PRESCRIPTIONS

A pharmacist must always be on guard for fake prescriptions. These can be

184

either written or called in by telephone.

Although coming across fake prescriptions is not a rare event, it's still an annoyance and something that pharmacists would rather not have to deal with.

My most memorable story was when a couple of guys came in and were laughing, joking and having a good time with our pharmacy intern as he took in their prescription. (People with fake prescriptions can often be over-friendly). The intern typed it up and filled it, yet when it came across my counter I could see that it was an obvious fake.

The funny part is that I was only a year or so out of pharmacy school. I was young looking, my hair was big and I didn't look much like a pharmacist, whereas the intern looked more distinguished and wore glasses. So I'm certain that the guys with the fake prescription felt they had won over the boss in charge.

I called the doctor who confirmed the prescription was a fake, and then I called the police. The two guys had been waiting in the lobby for at least 30 minutes, when suddenly they both jumped up and bolted to their car, almost like their intuition warned them to *GET OUT!!*

We watched out the window as rushed to their car. Suddenly, with a sudden change of heart, they talked themselves out of the fear and returned to the pharmacy. They waited for another ten minutes and then police came and arrested them.

*Another reminder to listen when your higher self is talking to you!*

That was the only time I ever called the police on a fake prescription. Generally pharmacists would rather have the people who write fake prescriptions just go away because turning them in will only add extra work.

Finally, a trick I learned from a pharmacist coworker: if you feel that the person on the phone is claiming to be a doctor and calling in a fake prescription, a good trick is to ask them for advice on a new drug that really doesn't exist, and listen as they squirm or hang up.

## MEDI-CAL FRAUD

Another aspect of thievery comes in the form of medical insurance fraud. This rampant system-wide corruption is often at the expense of taxpayers, since it is tax dollars that pay for both the services provided and the medications prescribed. Whether its practitioners double-billing or patients faking illness in order to receive free drugs, the system is severely flawed—top to bottom.

## WASTE OF MONEY

Medi-Cal is the state sponsored insurance that provides access to medical care and prescriptions for low income and uninsured residents. It has the best intentions for California's less fortunate inhabitants. But the system is broken, and patients are often medicated well beyond their actual need. To simplify, the patients only want drugs that are covered completely by insurance. Drug companies will jump through hoops to get their drug covered by Medi-Cal. The pharmaceutical companies are the ones who benefit the most making huge profits, while the patient gets whatever medication is covered. Once again, the individual's health is managed according to cost benefit, rather than health and wellness improvement. Consider these further examples of Medi-Cal's guidelines that generate huge expense for the state, and equivalent revenue streams to drug manufacturers:

1. Brand name drugs vs. generic – Insurance reimbursement guidelines demand that, when available, prescriptions are filled using generics over brand name medications. Some insurance plans allow brand name drugs, but the patient pays the price difference. This makes sense, and it does save money. Most patients who have insurance will receive a generic version of their drug when possible.

   However, there is an exception to this rule now, and the State (taxpayers) will reimburse certain prescriptions *only if* name brand is used. For example, a prescription for the antidepressant Prozac must be filled with the brand name version of the drug,

AND the State will pay an additional $110 over a generic version. Why does this happen? Drug companies point some of their profits to the State's General Fund. At least that is the explanation that I was given. Is this truly optimal use of taxpayer dollars?

The list of *name-brand only* is always evolving. Here are a few examples:

*Augmentin 500mg #20, which is an antibiotic commonly used for infections*
    *Brand: $165.99*
    *Generic: $78.99*
*Zithromax 200mg/5ml suspension 15ml, a commonly prescribed antibiotic in liquid form*
    *Brand: $73.99*
    *Generic: $34.99*
*Ortho Tri Cylen Lo, a birth control pill*
    *Brand: $49.99*
    *Generic: $32.99*
*Ortho Micronor, another birth control pill*
    *Brand: $59.99*
    *Generic: $38.99*
*Flonase Nasal Spray, a steroidal anti-inflammatory nasal spray for allergies*
    *Brand: $123.99*
    *Generic: $71.99*

2. Pharmacists waste amazing amounts of time every day calling doctors and insurance providers to clarify which drugs are covered and which are not. Each insurer has different guidelines, causing complication and wasted time. These guidelines change often as well, sometime annually, depending on what types of deals the insurance companies can make with the pharmaceutical companies.

## RX vs. OTC – ANOTHER WASTE OF MONEY

My next pet peeve in pharmacy-land is the cost difference between prescription (Rx) and over-the-counter (OTC) medications that provide the same remedy.

Let's review a couple of classics:

**The class of drug is known as Proton Pump Inhibitors (a.k.a. antacids).** Prevacid and Aciphex are prescription versions that cost $150 to $200 per month. Prilosec is over-the-counter, and costs approximately $30 per month. All three drugs work in the same fashion, and have a similar side effect profile. Why the difference in price? Because the prescription versions have a chance to be paid for by insurance, and the drug companies will get close to their asking price.

- Even though a drug is prescription, the insurance company picks up the tab and the patient is only responsible to pay a small $10 or $20 copay.
- With over the counter medications, a patient must pay the entire price, possibly $30.

So a $200 prescription medication costs less for the patient than a similar $30 over-the-counter medication. Again, these drugs are of the same class and therefore work the same with similar side effects.

**Claritin versus Clarinex.** Both are extremely similar in remedy and possible side effects. Over-the-counter Claritin will costs a buyer $30 for one month supply, verses $140 for prescription-only Clarinex. Insurance, especially Medi-Cal, will cover the higher-priced choice.

## CONTINUING EDUCATION

Pharmacists have Continuing Education (CE) requirements to fulfill every two years. Up to thirty units of CE provide information on the latest drugs to come onto the market among other topics of interest for pharmacists. Drug manufacturers offer these study guides and seminars free of charge, and most pharmacists will opt for the free CE credits. Thus, a pharmacist's continued awareness of drug trends is biased, to the point that there is a potential conflict of interest. Did I mention that dinner at a nice restaurant is included with these CE classes?

## CYCLE OF WASTE

There is one final aspect to my disdain of pharmacy: The Cycle of Waste. Millions, possibly billions, of dollars are spent each month for drugs and medications prescribed to people unnecessarily. It's a blatant fact that better health and wellness can occur by simply altering lifestyle, by improving attitude and eating habits. But then what would happen to the *business* of health insurance? We are led and trapped into the notion that paying money to insure our health is the best and only way. When will this spell be broken?

Patients want a medication that is covered by insurance. The pharmaceutical companies know this and work to get their drugs covered by as many insurance companies as possible. Even if doctors don't want to prescribe a drug, patients can be demanding and feel ripped off when leaving a doctor's office without a prescription. Now the doctors have devolved into a profession where healthcare is the ability to prescribe a drug covered on insurance. None of it has much to do with good health.

As I understand it, the basic premise of insurance—auto, home, life, but not health—is to provide financial protection against losses in case of accident or emergency, in exchange for a premium. What if you never got regular maintenance for your car, and then relied on insurance to pay monthly for tape on the engine, or to change the patch on the tires? The health insurance swindle extracts money from a person every month in order to pay for maintenance of poor lifestyle habits. When an actual emergency arises, insurance companies do everything in their power *not to pay*. This is why a leading cause of bankruptcy in America is due to overwhelming medical bills, when a person's *health insurance runs out*.

## SUMMARY

The pharmacy profession used to be about health. In the old days, the pharmacist would be knowledgeable of natural remedies, and simple solutions to health problems. Now the profession has devolved far away from patient health and the pharmacist is only trained with the knowledge that will create profits for pharmaceutical companies.

Imagine spending your days running around a monkey cage, dealing with the sick and impatient customers, answering to the many authorities, trying to protect the inventory from a variety of thieves, and identifying fraudulent prescriptions. All in effort to provide medications that often aren't improving the patient's health and that are being prescribed for conditions that can be treated by better methods.

## POINTS TO REMEMBER:

- I don't like pharmacy.

- Drugs are covered on health plans because insurance companies make deals with the pharmaceutical companies, not because they are the best options for healthcare.

- Pharmacists have become a powerless pawn in the big world of pharmaceutical profits.

## INTERVIEW WITH TOURETTE'S SYNDROME DEFEATER AND WELLNESS COACH/FITNESS TRAINER FRANK TORTORICI

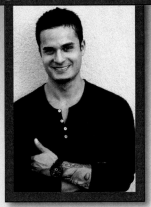

*Frank Tortorici grew up in Long Island, New York. As a child, he struggled with Tourette' syndrome. Frank tried pharmaceuticals to treat the symptoms without success. In 7th grade, he started to train with weights. He discovered working out had a calming effect on him. He also noticed when exercising his symptoms caused by Tourette syndrome were lessened. He later learned that bodybuilding wasn't nearly as healthy as it appeared, as participants often used unhealthy or unnatural products and steroids. As a result, he started to learn about natural ways to eat and then natural ways to treat Tourette syndrome. Frank now works as a counselor and personal trainer to teach his clients a more natural and sustainable way of health.*

**Dr. Leyla: What was your life like as a child?**
Frank: I came from a loving family. I had a great support system and I was one of the star pitchers on the baseball team in elementary school.

**Dr. Leyla: When did you start noticing symptoms of Tourette syndrome?**
Frank: It all started in 3rd grade. I started noticing symptoms in high pressure situations, such as blinking of the eyes, head snapping, and I would make squeaky noises. My stomach would distend, and I would hear noises like the sound of water movement in a water bed. Other symptoms were more subtle—I would make funny faces, or if I were on a treadmill my knees would bang together. At first it seemed like a nervous habit. After a certain point, I was diagnosed with Tourette syndrome.

**Dr. Leyla: How did it affect your life?**
Frank: It was difficult to visit quiet places because I never knew when it

191

would flare up. In school, when it was time to take tests the room was quiet and I would have to focus on masking symptoms. I avoided libraries and movie theaters. It created a lot of embarrassment and pain because I never knew when the symptoms would appear.

**Dr. Leyla: What do you think is the cause of the Tourette syndrome?**
Frank: The doctors will tell you that the cause is unknown, or attribute it to a disorder in the brain. I believe that it's a toxicity issue. I had lots of vaccinations growing up. Also, I grew up in Long Island which has the highest rate of breast cancer. There are also other people there with Tourette syndrome. I had allergies severe enough that I had to get allergy shots once a week for years. Additionally, my mother delivered me by C-section, and I wasn't breast fed, so I had a weakened immune system. I don't think there is a single cause, but I believe all these factors add up to a condition.

**Dr. Leyla: What types of medications were prescribed to you?**
Frank: Haloperidol was the first drug, but it caused insomnia and shortness of breath. The doctors were always trying to push another drug. After a few drugs that didn't work and caused side effects, my parents became more and more hesitant to put drugs down my throat.

**Dr. Leyla: When did things change?**
Frank: I started working out and training with weights in 7th grade. I went hard core at the gym and I competed in body building contests in 9th and 11th grade. I learned discipline but I also learned when I was concentrating on something or focused, then the symptoms faded. Still today when I'm training, exercising, or writing, or in a zone of some kind—fixated on something—then the symptoms are lessened.

**Dr. Leyla: Did the body building cure your condition?**
Frank: From that point I got passionate about bodybuilding as there were pro-amateur body builders in my gym. However, that's when I learned body building was actually very unhealthy. There was a lot of drug and steroid abuse going on. From age 16 until age 21 I was in a very dark, dark part of my life with alcohol and recreational drugs. I

tried steroids, but only for a week or so. I was on heavy protein shakes, protein bars, and my ticks were getting worse. It took lots of unhealthy habits to get to the point of competing in a body building competition.

**Dr. Leyla: When did your life changed?**
Frank: In December 1999 I had a major turning point when lots of people who I thought were close friends got arrested for selling steroids and drugs. I was devastated as to how quickly they all changed to save their own butts, and I learned situations like that are an opportunity to learn who your true friends really are.

And then in June 2000 I had another moment. I was at an audition when the symptoms really started to flare up. I was auditioning with another actor and there were 3 or 4 casting agents at the table. My body felt out of control as my head was shaking, my stomach was making gurgling sounds, and my body was twitching. Because I was so self-conscious of my body I couldn't remember any of my lines. I just remembered the looks on their faces, the energy in the room, and the uncomfortable silence. Needless to say, I bombed the audition.

**Dr. Leyla: What did that mean for you?**
Frank: At that time in my life I was taking lots of painkillers, muscle relaxers, and drinking alcohol. That moment was a turning point for me, when I realized I had hit rock bottom and I had to make some changes.

**Dr. Leyla: How did your life change?**
Frank: This time was the start of a rebirthing process for me. I gave up the recreational drugs and any abuse of my body and I went from a heavy meat eater to a raw and vegetarian lifestyle. I also adopted a gluten-free diet and tried different ways to see how the symptoms would respond. I tried to eat from the purest sources possible, and switched to food based supplements, with a whole food based diet. I researched how to treat Tourette syndrome holistically, and I learned how sugar and alcohol can attribute to the symptoms. This is the time when I became spiritually enlightened as well. I learned Buddhism, and I fell in love with the Agape International Spiritual Center.

Sometimes you have to hit rock bottom to be victorious.

**Dr. Leyla: How are you helping others with Tourette syndrome?**
Frank: I've spoken at the Tourette Syndrome Association (TSA) conference and shared my experience and success with Tourette syndrome. I'm letting people know as much as possible that there is much more than what doctors will tell you or prescribe for you.

**Dr. Leyla: What advice would you give to athletes?**
Frank: There is really nothing healthy about extreme competitive sports or body building. Being a professional athlete requires an abnormal obsession of food, heavy protein, and heavy lifting which is not natural. These habits eventually take a toll on the body, especially body builders. Often professional athletes are expected to perform at any expense, and as a result many take enhancement drugs, steroids, pain killers, cortisone shots to the knees or lower back, often playing while still injured— doing whatever is necessary to keep up their performance. All these things cause damage later, which is the price they pay to be professional athletes. Yet the wear and tear their bodies go through is tremendous and they will be paying the price for many years later. If they would put good nutrients in their bodies, and allow their bodies to heal and repair itself when necessary, they would have greater health and longevity.

**Dr. Leyla: What services do you provide?**
Frank: Right now I'm working with a service I call Extreme Makeover. This includes functional fitness, functional diagnostic nutrition, and adaptation of spiritual practices (meditations, affirmations, and self-help books). I also offer a test in which I am certified to read hormone levels, cortisol, and liver detox. We take a saliva sample and send it to the laboratory. Then the results provide a nutritional interpretation which is like a blueprint on how to change your life.

**Dr. Leyla: Do you have a favorite success story to share?**
Frank: I have had many great stories over the years, but the one that stands out the most was a client I had in New York. She came to me 125 pounds overweight, a smoker, and a major sweet tooth. She hated

exercise and was in a constant battle with depression. After six months of training together, she dropped the 125 pounds, quit smoking, and got so inspired she quit her job as a nurse and became a certified trainer.

**Dr. Leyla: What is your mission?**
Frank: My mission now is to do whatever I can to assist people in realizing they can unlock their god-given potential. I like to work on people with the mind, body, and soul; and I like to work with food, and spiritual principles including training and nutritional counseling. I'm also dedicated to keeping my body in the best shape I can. If I can't live it then I shouldn't teach it.

**Dr. Leyla: What would be your message to the world?**
Frank: I would tell people to start learning how to eat intuitively, and not fall prey to the drug companies and corporate advertising. Food truly is medicine, and when we bring it back to basics, and eat what god intended, we will receive all the benefits of a healthy and vital lifestyle.

Eating cleaner food sources will allow your thinking to be clearer. With this new level of clarity you can see through all the smoke and mirrors of the corruption that is going on. You understand better, especially with health issues, when the media tells you to go left, you should go right. When one person makes that shift, then the family and those surrounding them will see the benefits and also be more likely to make changes.

As the late Tupac Shakur once said,

"I don't plan on changing the world, but I plan on sparking the brain cells of those that will."

**Frank Tortorici**
**(323) 839-0868**

**FrankTortorici.com**

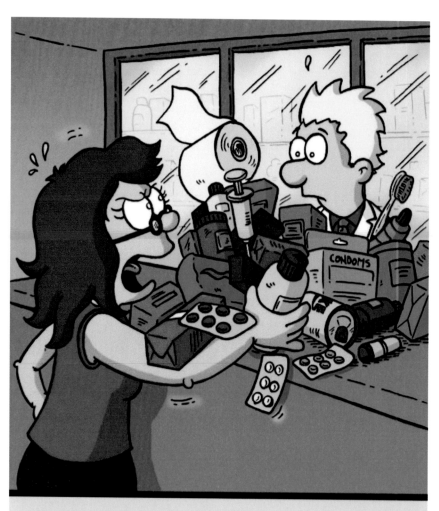

$10??!! WHADDAYAMEAN?? I HAVE INSURANCE!

## CHAPTER 12

# CASE STUDY

*The best doctor gives the least medicines.*
*~Benjamin Franklin*

This section is a case study of a 54-year old female patient from a pharmacy in Los Angeles, California. For privacy purposes, she is referred to as *Patient Abigail.* Although the patient's list of medications is a more extreme example, it shows what can become of patients who rely solely on a medical doctor to treat health conditions.

## MEDICATIONS

Here is a description of Patient Abigail's monthly medications. (See table 12.1)

**Medications (#1-11)** are for diabetes. Actos,[154] glyburide and metformin[155] are all tablets that lower blood sugar levels. Novolog is short-acting insulin to be used with each meal,[156] while Lantus is long-acting insulin used once-a-day,[157] and Lantus Solostar is an easy-to-use pre-filled syringe for patient convenience.[158] To round out the list of injectable medications, Byetta "may improve blood sugar control in adults . . . when used with a diet and exercise program."[159] In addition to medication, most diabetics will need syringes, test strips, lancets, and alcohol swabs on a monthly basis.

Total cost for her diabetes care: $1,302 per month.

**Medications (#12-14)** Norvasc, doxazosin, and labetalol help lower blood pressure.

**Medications (#15-17)** Metolazone, spironolactone, and furosemide are diuretics to deal with fluid retention.

**Potassium (#18)** must be added to the mix to replace the lost potassium. A side effect of the diuretic furosemide causes loss of potassium.

**Clarinex (#19)** is for nasal allergies. It is similar to the over-the-counter Claritin.[160]

**Nitroglycerin (#20)** is to be used if Patient Abigail experiences chest pain, angina, or other symptoms of a heart attack. It works quickly to increase blood flow to the heart by dilating the blood vessels surrounding the heart.[161]

**Aciphex (#21)** is used to reduce acid in the stomach.[162]

**Clonazepam (#22)** is used to reduce anxiety or as a sleep aid.[163]

**Celebrex (#23)** is for pain, swelling and stiffness due to certain arthritic conditions.[164]

**Calcium (#24)** and **Ferrous Sulfate (Iron, #25)** are given when the patient's level of these are deficient.

**Vicodin (#26)** is used to reduce moderate or severe pain, with constipation as one of the side effects.[165]

**Docusate Sodium (#27)** is a stool softener to help manage, or prevent constipation.[166]

**Diphenhydramine (Benadryl) (#28)** is for allergies, and often used as a sleep aid.

**Vytorin (#29)** is a combination pill to manage cholesterol levels, which works to lower *bad cholesterol* and raise *good cholesterol*.[167]

**198**

**Temazepam (#30)** is a sleeping pill.[168]

**Promethazine with codeine (#31)** is an addictive narcotic cough syrup.[169]

**Procrit (#32)** is a biotech drug used for anemia.[170]

**Geodon (#33)** and **Abilify (#34)** are newer antipsychotic medications.[171,172]

**Flonase (#35)** is a steroidal anti-inflammatory nose spray for allergies.[173]

**Medications (#36-41)** Spiriva, theophylline, Singulair, Xopenex inhaler, Xopenex solution, and ipratroprium bromide are all for breathing and respiratory problems, including asthma and Chronic Obstructive Pulmonary Disease (COPD).

### Important Notes regarding Patient Abigail

1. Patient is prescribed Clarinex (#19) every month, which carries a $145 monthly cost. Claritin is an over-the-counter and equally effective alternative, which costs $30 per month. Why is Patient Abigail taking the more expensive version? It's simply a matter of which drug is *covered* by her health insurance; for her, it's *free*.

2. Patient Abigail is on two brand medications, Norvasc (#12) and Flonase (#35). The state will only cover the brand name versions of these, even though a generic is available.

   Total extra cost per month: $147.

3. Spiriva (#36) and ipratropium (#41) are used to tackle Chronic Obstructive Pulmonary Disease (COPD),[174] which is often a direct result of being a smoker.

4. The total cost of Patient Abigail's medications is **$5,747 per month.**

   Where does the money come from? Since her medications are covered by the state's Medi-Cal plan, it is the people of

California—the taxpayers—who are paying to maintain this monthly drug regimen. She doesn't pay a penny.

5. Diabetes sufferers are top-level customers to the pharmaceutical industry. As their condition worsens the drug regimen usually progresses, and these medications are almost always covered by insurance plans.

Although Abigail's situation may be extreme, it is not completely rare. Often patients are willing to take whatever the doctor recommends as long as it is covered by insurance. There are millions of people taking too much medication and it is not restoring their health, only maintaining poor health.

Also to note, most cases of type 2 diabetes can be completely reversed in a matter of weeks with a change in diet and lifestyle.

## LESSONS LEARNED

Abigail's profile is shown to demonstrate:

1. The excessive use of drugs.
2. The excessive cost of drugs.
3. Drugs are a successful business system.
4. Most of these conditions are preventable.
5. Abigail goes to her doctor, covered by her insurance, and is prescribed medications, also covered by her insurance. Her insurance dictates her healthcare regimen.
6. Abigail is a true example of *Off Balance, The American Way of Health*.

Table 12.1
*Patient Abigail's monthly medications*

| Medication | Dosage | Quantity | Monthly Cost ($) |
|---|---|---|---|
| 1. Actos | 45mg | 30 | 250 |
| 2. Glyburide | 5mg | 120 | 72 |
| 3. Metformin | 500mg | 60 | 30 |
| 4. Novolog | 100 u/ml vial | 10 ml | 103 |
| 5. Lantus | 100 u/ml vial | 20 ml | 202 |
| 6. Lantus Solostar | 100 u/ml vial | 15 ml | 210 |
| 7. Byetta | 10mcg inj | 2 | 280 |
| 8. Syringes | | 100 | 32 |
| 9. Test Strips | | 100 | 102 |
| 10. Lancets | | 100 | 18 |
| 11. Alcohol swabs | | 100 | 3 |
| | | | |
| 12. Norvasc | 10mg | 30 | 102 ($75) |
| 13. Doxazosin | 4mg | 90 | 95 |
| 14. Labetalol | 300mg | 90 | 93 |
| 15. Metolazone | 5mg | 30 | 54 |
| 16. Spironolactone | 25mg | 60 | 32 |
| 17. Furosemide | 80mg | 90 | 25 |
| 18. Potassium Liquid | 10% | 960 ml | 15 |
| | | | |
| 19. Clarinex | 5mg | 30 | 145 |
| 20. Nitroglycerin | 0.4mg SL | 100 | 15 |
| 21. Aciphex | 20mg | 30 | 220 |
| 22. Clonazepam | 1mg | 60 | 48 |
| 23. Celebrex | 200mg | 60 | 255 |
| 24. Calcium | 500mg | 60 | 7 |
| 25. Ferrous Sulfate | 325mg | 100 | 10 |
| 26. Vicodin | | 60 | 33 |
| 27. Docusate Sodium | 100mg | 100 | 11 |
| 28. Diphenhydramine | 25mg | 30 | 5 |
| 29. Vytorin | 10-40mg | 30 | 210 |
| 30. Temazepam | 30mg | 30 | 21 |
| 31. Promethazine/cod | 480ml | | 42 |
| 32. Procrit | 10,000 u/ml vial | 6 | 990 |

**201**

| Medication | Dosage | Quantity | Monthly Cost ($) |
|---|---|---|---|
| 33. Geodon | 60mg | 90 | 795 |
| 34. Abilify | 30mg | 30 | 375 |
| 35. Flonase nasal spray | 16ml | | 110 ($72) |
| 36. Spiriva | 18mcg | 30 | 182 |
| 37. Theophylline | 200mg | 120 | 36 |
| 38. Singulair | 10mg | 30 | 138 |
| 39. Xopenex Inhaler | 15ml | | 112 |
| 40. Xopenex Solution vials | 144ml | | 199 |
| 41. Ipratropium Bromide | 75ml | | 70 |

**Is this the best form of healthcare? Or even the cheapest?**

It's not cheap, and its' not health. In fact, if Abigail had to pay for her monthly medication regimen, chances are she would look to see what other types of healthcare are available. But this is what the doctors and so-called experts recommend to Abigail. This is the norm in American society. It's simply too convenient. It's a hype that has veered dreadfully out of control.

## WHAT CAN BE DONE INSTEAD?

Alternative healthcare options could benefit health and save money. Why doesn't this happen? Again, the people who have the money make the rules. Alternative healthcare options are often not covered by insurance, and are therefore much more expensive for the patient.

**Would it be possible to reduce the number of Abigail's medications?**

The answer is, definitively, YES!

**Type 2 Diabetes:** Abigail's diabetes medications cost the taxpayers $1,303 per month. Yet, type 2 diabetes is a simple condition.

For a quick review of type 2 diabetes, sugar is eaten and digested and then taken by the bloodstream to the cells where it is used for energy. With

**202**

excess sugar intake, the cells are now overloaded with sugar which creates insulin resistance, causing the cells to reject the excess sugar. The sugar then remains in the bloodstream. However, the blood cannot hold excessive sugar or will get too thick. Therefore, fluid must now move from the cells to the bloodstream to compensate for this excess sugar.

The essence of diabetic medications is to reduce the level of sugar in the bloodstream. Often, the medications work to push the sugar into cells somehow, as well as other mechanisms of action, and then the glucose test improves. However, the diabetic drugs will never get a patient with insulin resistance to a healthier or more balanced state. The only real solution is to stop eating excessive amounts of sugar.

The fact is type 2 diabetes is easy to reverse with a natural and unprocessed foods diet.[175] It may be difficult for many, as eating this food can be more expensive, much less convenient and feel less emotionally satisfying. However, diabetes is a simple disease with a simple solution. No pill will ever cure type 2 diabetes by shoving excess sugar from the blood into a cell.

**Respiratory conditions:** Abigail is on seven medications for asthma, including one for chronic obstructive pulmonary disease, which causes the lungs to lose elasticity, and is often associated with smoking.[176] We cannot be certain whether or not Abigail is or was a smoker, but it is very likely.

In the world of doctors and drugs, asthma is a chronic disease for which there is no cure. In the holistic world, there are people that have been healed through cleansing and modification of diet. Asthma is often caused by swelling in the lungs, and swelling indicates that there is something in the lungs that the body is trying to get out.

**Blood Pressure:** Abigail is also taking seven medications for blood pressure. These could also be eliminated or reduced with a change in diet and lifestyle. Often patients are told they will be on blood pressure medications for the rest of their lives, but that also does not have to be true as it can be treated by a variety of holistic practitioners.

**Cholesterol and Stomach Acid:** Abigail is taking Vytorin and Aciphex for these conditions. Together the two drugs costs over $450 per month, and can easily be eliminated with a natural and unprocessed food diet.

**Anxiety and Insomnia:** Abigail is taking Clonazepam for anxiety. Temazepam and diphenhydramine are both for sleep. There are holistic practices that have calming effects on patients, such as breathing exercises, meditation, relaxation techniques, and by using the power of the mind.[177,178]

For Abigail, going to the doctor and picking up a bunch of medications is, unfortunately, the path of least resistance.

If Abigail chooses to take action in attempt to stop taking at least some of her medications, she would have to be proactive, and go beyond society's norm for healthcare. Fast food and drugs are the most convenient options in our world today, but they are nothing more than a quick and convenient alternative to better choices. Abigail would need the desire to change, learn how to eat properly, and learn other holistic practices that can help her live a healthier, happier and drug-free lifestyle.

**POINTS TO REMEMBER:**

- If you are compliant, and follow the directions of your doctor and pharmacist, you may wind up with a boatload of medications all covered by health insurance, but remain in very poor health.

## INTERVIEW WITH *MAY I BE FRANK'S* FRANK FERRANTE

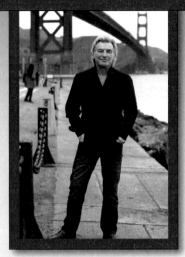

*Frank Ferrante, was a Sicilian from Brooklyn living in San Francisco. He was morbidly obese, pre-diabetic, and fighting Hepatitis C. At age 54 his transformational journey started when he walked into Café Gratitude, a raw food restaurant in San Francisco. He got to know the three guys who worked there and shared with them his struggles with his health. They decided to assist Frank with his transformation. Frank openly shares his journey to health in his documentary movie "May I Be Frank".*

**Dr. Leyla: What was your life like before your transformation?**
Frank: I was fat, angry and tired all the time. I was lonely, dismal, depressed. I was divorced with two grown kids. But I was estranged from my daughter and that caused me lots of pain.

**Dr. Leyla: How was your health?**
Frank: I was 100 pounds overweight. I was pre-diabetic and I had hepatitis C. And I was tired all the time. To further complicate matters, I didn't know why I was tired. I wondered if it was from the hepatitis, or from the medication, or from some other reason. I didn't know why I felt so bad.

**Dr. Leyla: What types of medications were you on?**
Frank: I took a handful of medications. I didn't know what everything was, but I had Lipitor for my cholesterol which was over 300. I took Effexor for depression and Celebrex for joint pain. I also took Interferon and Ribavarin, which are strong medications for hepatitis C, and they caused lots of side effects.

**Dr. Leyla: How did the medical treatment affect your health?**
Frank: I felt terrible all the time. The problem was that every time a new symptom or problem would come up, the doctor would treat it with another prescription and another pill. It felt like they were just piling them on with no other solution, and no end in sight.

**Dr. Leyla: Did you feel let down, or disappointed by your medical doctor and the drugs?**
Frank: Yes. Another problem is that I was a former alcoholic and drug addict. The doctors had no concept of drug addiction. They gave me Vicodin, which is a narcotic. I knew it was going to be a problem, but when I expressed that to the doctor he didn't seem to get it. He said just take the amount written on the bottle and then you won't have a problem. But addicts don't do that. And I knew I was in trouble when I was watching the clock waiting for the time to take the next pill.

**Dr. Leyla: Were you able to control that?**
Frank: For a while, but eventually it spiraled out of control. I was soon seeing multiple doctors and going to different pharmacies to get more of the drug.

**Dr. Leyla: What was rock bottom for you? When did you decide to change your life?**
Frank: I knew my life could be much, much better, but I had no idea how to do it or where to start. But I knew that something needed to change, and I needed a shift.

**Dr. Leyla: Then what happened?**
Frank: The movie tells the story, but I walked into a raw food restaurant in San Francisco called Café Gratitude. I started talking with some of the boys that worked there. I told them about my situation, and from there they decided they would help me with my transformation.

**Dr. Leyla: What did the transformation consist of?**
Frank: I committed to turning my life over to the three young men (all in their twenties) who were going to help me physically, emotionally and spiritually for the next 42 days.

**206**

**Dr. Leyla: What did the program include?**
Frank: There was a lot to it. It consisted of change in food, workbooks, affirmations, colonics, and daily exercise. I ate raw and vegan food, and I drank wheat grass and water. On a physical level, I committed to walking 15 minutes every day. And on the emotional level I did affirmations and I was also able to mend the relationship with my daughter.

**Dr. Leyla: What food was included in your meals?**
Frank: Every day I ate three meals at Café Gratitude which consisted of raw, vegan, organic food. For breakfast I had four ounces of wheatgrass and a 16-ounce smoothie (coconut milk, figs, cacao, blue green algae, vanilla, dates, Himalayan salt and ice). For lunch I had a raw sunflower seed based enchilada with spinach tortilla served with a salad with tahini dressing with a 16-ounce green juice (cucumber, celery, kale and lemon). And for dinner a large Café Salad mixed greens, shredded carrots, beets, cucumbers, sunflower sprouts, avocado, brazil nut "parmesan," a flax carrot cracker and tahini dressing. Also every day I drink one gallon of water.

**Dr. Leyla: What was the physical commitment?**
Frank: In the beginning, I rode the bicycle at the gym for only five minutes and I would be completely winded. But I committed to walking every day for 15 minutes. Then I went to the gym where I met people who were encouraging and it felt more comfortable.

**Dr. Leyla: What types of affirmations?**
Frank: I would look in the mirror and say things like "I am beautiful" and "I am radiant health." At first they were very hard to say because when you're looking at yourself while saying the affirmations you feel like a liar. In the past I would use self-deprecating humor as a way to cope with being overweight. I would call myself a "fat bastard." But I committed to stopping that. One day a friend told me that if he heard someone talking to me the way I was talking to myself then he would kick their ass. That got to me and I understood what he meant. People have a resistance to saying beautiful things about themselves. But I learned if you want something you never had, you have to so do something that you've never done.

**Dr. Leyla: Besides food and exercise, what else was part of your commitment and transformation?**

Frank: Those were the main things, but there was actually much more to it. I visited a holistic practitioner, I did some workbooks, I went to a yoga retreat and learned some meditations. I also worked on dealing with emotions that I hadn't dealt with and let go of some pain and anger that I was holding on to. There was also a very spiritual part to it.

**Dr. Leyla: What is the main lesson?**

Frank: I think the first thing is learning to love yourself. It's about doing things to take care of yourself and talking to yourself in a way that is self-empowering and loving.

**Dr. Leyla: Was it all uphill after the 42 days? Did it get easier?**

Frank: No, actually after the 42 days I lost contact with the boys and went the other direction. I was back on the pain pills and reconnected with my addictive tendencies. I almost died at one point before I returned to doing the right things.

**Dr. Leyla: There are lots of people currently struggling with their health, similar to your previous situation and health. What is the difference between you and the others who haven't gone through a transformation?**

Frank: There really is no difference. There is nothing special about me. It just takes a willingness to move forward and make the steps. You can have all the knowledge, but if you're not willing to take the steps it doesn't do any good. But trust me, if I can do this then anyone can. And it's amazing the people that show up in your life when you are honest with yourself and open and willing to receiving help.

**Dr. Leyla: And how is your life now? Do you continue a strict raw food diet and exercise regimen?**

Frank: I've lost about 120 pounds and I've gotten off of all medications. I don't just eat raw foods. I certainly have a large portion of my diet from natural and healthy sources. But it's really not as much about the food as it is about loving yourself and doing the things to take care of yourself. I used to love eating cheesecake, but now it doesn't appeal to me, mostly because after I eat it I don't feel good. I also work out in the gym four to five times per week.

**Dr. Leyla: What would your message be to those who want to follow your path and transform their lives?**
Frank: It's really about discovering self-love. When you discover that, it's amazing what comes into your life.

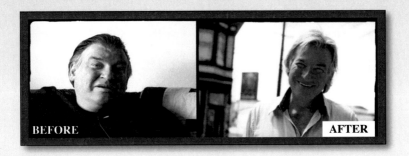

**Frank Ferrante**

**MayIBeFrankMovie.com**

209

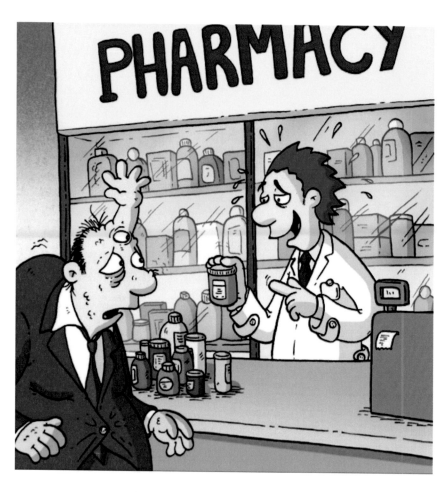

OOPS... SORRY,
JUST TAKE THESE TO
MAKE THAT GO AWAY.

CHAPTER 13

# ARE DRUGS REALLY A PROBLEM?

*We sometimes joke that when you're doing a clinical trial, there are two possible disasters. The first disaster is if you kill people. The second disaster is if you cure them. The truly good drugs are the ones you can use chronically over a long, long time.*
*~Alex Hittle, a biotech analyst at AG Edwards in St Louis*

All businesses have to make money. Healthcare in our society is a business. A patient gets sick, and then goes to his doctor, who provides a service by guiding and assisting the patient to get well. At least that's how it used to be. How did the healthcare system end up so far down the wrong path?

## THE BUSINESS OF DRUGS

Historically, many health solutions have come about via the industry of producing drugs. At some point a gradual shift occurred in the American medical evolution, and the intentions turned away from achieving optimal health and wellness and towards a business of earning money. However, the profits are not earned by providing good health services, but rather, *at the expense of patient's good health.*

Collectively, we have developed into a society which profits on our physical and mental ailments. Stockholders invest in business that make money. Pharmaceutical salespeople want recognition and a nice bonus, while doctors and pharmacists enjoy prestige and the perks offered by the drug companies, like free dinners and sponsored trips wrapped around a convention promoting drug solutions. (Although there are new laws requiring drug companies to report any payments to physicians).[179] Lastly, the patients are seeking health in a pill—a quick fix. So really, everyone is happy. Who's complaining?

However, there's a big problem. The quest for profit far overrides the quest for health and wellness, at a level if many fully understood they would be shocked, even sickened.

Here are some problems that are discussed in this chapter:

- Drugs are promoted when there are simpler, less expensive holistic solutions.

- Drugs are covered by insurance, while holistic solutions are not.

- Patients want drugs.

- Doctors are mostly trained in prescribing drugs.

- Insurance companies determine which drugs are covered on the health plan. If a medication is covered, it is then affordable for the patient.

- Drugs are advertised directly to the general public. Patients will then ask their doctor to write a prescription for that drug.

- Drugs are promoted to appeal to children.

- Errors caused by drugs result in many deaths each year.

- Adverse effects from taking drugs correctly, as prescribed, also cause harm and sometimes death to patients.

- New problems and side effects are discovered a few years after a drug is sold on the market.

- The making of a drug has become almost a joke, filled with exaggerations, misrepresentations, and plain lies.

- The Food and Drug Administration (FDA) no longer has the consumer's good health as their first priority.

212

- Even when a drug causes harm to patients and the drug company must pay a settlement, the amount they have to pay hardly creates a dent in their massive profits.

- Drug companies are not interested in drugs that will cure a condition; they are interested in long-term use and profits.

- The healthcare system has become automated and impersonal, and disconnected from the human touch of healing.

As a result, the entire healthcare system has become a ridiculous circus of people running in circles following rules and regulations, while the population gets sicker and the pharmaceutical companies get richer.

## DRUGS ARE PROMOTED WHEN THERE ARE SIMPLER, LESS EXPENSIVE HOLISTIC SOLUTIONS.

Expensive medications are often used for the stomach when simpler, natural solutions exist. Nexium suppresses acid in the stomach and is used for heartburn. In 2011, Nexium was the third highest-selling drug, earning over five billion dollars in sales. Lipitor, which reduces cholesterol levels, came in first as the highest-selling drug with over seven billion dollars in sales.[180]

Both of these drugs could easily be discontinued by patients changing their diets.

That is also the case with many other top sellers. There are holistic and natural remedies for many common health conditions that are routinely treated with expensive pharmaceutical drugs.

## DRUGS ARE COVERED BY INSURANCE, WHILE HOLISTIC SOLUTIONS ARE NOT.

Big changes need to occur at this juncture. Insurance companies spend so much money to maintain poor health. Recently a growing number of insurance companies are willing to pay for certain holistic treatments, such as acupuncture and chiropractic. However, there's still a long way to go. Huge amounts of money are being spent on pharmaceuticals as patients continue to get sicker. Diabetic medications typically cost between $350 to $900 per month.[181]

What if that money was used instead to teach the patient to change their lifestyle, and to support and empower the patient in healing themselves through holistic means?

What if patients were financially rewarded for getting off expensive and ridiculous medications?

For example, Lipitor costs about $200 per month, or $2400 per year. The patients would be encouraged to get natural remedies for cholesterol, and change their lifestyle to get off the drug. Once the patient is off the medication, then they would be offered a financial incentive as a reward. The savings would be passed down to the patients.

Some of the interviews of previous chapters also demonstrate these absurd and unnecessary expenses of Western medicine. Here is a review of a few of them from previous chapters:

**Pain (Chapter 7 Interview)**
Art San had a motorcycle injury that lead to severe and chronic back pain. Doctors recommended surgery and said he should expect to have back pain the rest of his life. Although he refused the surgery, the costs could have been $10,000 to $20,000.

vs.

After twenty years of suffering, Art learned how to get himself out of pain by using muscle releasing techniques. Costs: Training in massage and acupressure points.

**Hepatitis B (Chapter 4 Interview)**
Former pharmacist Dr. Kinnane had a friend who was diagnosed with hepatitis B and went to a prestigious hospital for treatment. After one month

and over $150,000 in medical bills, he passed away.

vs.

A patient with hepatitis B walked in Dr. Kinnane's pharmacy, and Dr. Kinnane recommended dandelion root tea as a Chinese herbal remedy. The patient was relieved of all his symptoms in less than one month. Costs: price of tea approximately $5.

### Neuropathy (Chapter 8 Interview)
Duncan Tooley suffered for 3 years with neuropathy that was *incurable.* He received infusions of Gamma Globulin twice a month costing $10,000 each time. Annual cost: $240,000.

vs.

Duncan cured his own neuropathy with hypnotherapy. Costs: training sessions to become a hypnotherapist.

### Cancer (Chapter 10 Interview)
Susan Moss saw her friend go through chemotherapy, radiation, surgery and a bone marrow transplant. After over five years of pain and suffering, she passed away at age 38. Cost: Over $350,000.

vs.

When Susan was diagnosed with cancer she took the cancer into her own hands and used a variety of techniques, including cleansing, visualization, releasing of emotions, chanting and exercise. Costs: minimal, including natural foods and gym membership.

These are just a few examples of the amazing possibilities of healing.

*I believe there are affordable and natural solutions for every health condition.*

## PATIENTS WANT DRUGS

This is a huge problem and one I'm hoping this book will lead people to

**215**

think twice about. Drugs are recommended by respected professionals. They are in magazines, on television, and available at pharmacies on many corners. Patients feel if they have good insurance, then they're entitled to the newest and greatest drugs. The underlying belief is that drugs are a solution to the problem, and the key to good health. Yet this is rarely the case. This is merely a belief system that was created by the ones who hold the power and take control of our advertising, and therefore define what is acceptable or normal in our reality.

As a result, patients have become a big part of the problem. They don't go to the doctor seeking wellness information, or tips for a healthy lifestyle. They want drugs.

## DOCTORS ARE MOSTLY TRAINED IN PRESCRIBING DRUGS.

In the old days, doctors were trained more about health and less about drugs. Doctors would talk to their patients and get to know them. They would go to patients' houses, and tap on the knees to test the reflexes.

Today, doctors are minimally trained in nutrition. Doctors are not trained in how to identify toxins or remove them from the body. Additionally, they are not trained in how emotions can lead to physical conditions, and they definitely are not trained how to help the patients tap into their own healing powers.

Now doctors are trained only in drugs. During their training they are taught the holistic alternatives are inferior or even quackery. Nowadays you get ten minutes with your insurance approved doctor. If you're lucky you get a prescription, and if you're really lucky it's covered by insurance.

## INSURANCE COMPANIES DETERMINE WHICH DRUGS ARE COVERED ON THE HEALTHPLAN. IF A MEDICATION IS COVERED, THEN IT IS AFFORDABLE FOR THE PATIENT.

It used to be patients would be examined by their doctor, and the doctor would decide the course of treatment. If a patient's insurance plan does not pay for a drug, then often the patient cannot afford to pay for it either. Now the insurance companies determine standard accepted protocol for treatment. Doctors have less control over what they choose to prescribe for their patients.

## DRUGS ARE ADVERTISED DIRECTLY TO THE GENERAL PUBLIC. PATIENTS WILL THEN ASK THEIR DOCTOR TO WRITE A PRESCRIPTION FOR THAT DRUG.

Once upon a time the doctors were the ones who were most educated on drugs. When the patient came for an appointment, the doctor would recommend whatever therapy or drug he felt was best.

Direct-to-consumer advertising was legalized by the FDA in the 1990s.[182] This allows drug companies to appeal to the masses by advertising on television, on radio, in magazines, and on the internet. Now when a patient goes to the doctor, they want that colorful, fun-looking drug they saw on television—the drug that turned their television screen from black-and-white to color and happiness. Not only do doctors have insurance guidelines to live by, they also have patients requesting the newest fad drug being advertised. Will the doctors prescribe what their patients request?

In 2005, the drug companies spent $29.9 billion on direct-to-consumer advertising, leading to increase in sales and overuse of some medications.[183]

It's like putting colorful cereal boxes at a level where kids can reach and grab it. Then they tell their parents they want it. If they want the cereal bad enough, they'll ask for it, maybe even demand it. The more they demand it and the more they have a tantrum if they don't get it, the greater the cereal's sales and profit.[184] Except now the adults are the one who are demanding.

## DRUGS ARE PROMOTED TO APPEAL TO CHILDREN.

Drug companies create characters and stuffed animals to appeal to children.

**217**

**Digger**

Lamisil (terbinafine) is an antifungal used to treat toenail fungus. The nails become rough, discolored and weak. To appeal to children, *Digger* was created. Digger was a cute, ugly, animated yellow-gray monster that would appeal to children and make curing toenail fungus fun. Terbinafine was promoted to wipe out Digger. However, the treatment takes 6 weeks, and the FDA has put out a health advisory that terbinafine is toxic to the liver.[185]

**Sesame Street**

Zithromax is an antibiotic prescribed to children for ear infections. While showing images of children playing happily with a zebra and a giant colorful tumbling wooden block with the letter "Z" on its side, the voiceover reads "the show was made possible by a grant from Pfizer which. . . brings parents the letter Z, as in Zithromax."[186]

Sesame Street also had an episode featuring the furry red Elmo as he went to the doctor's office to treat his ear infection. The doctor examined Elmo and then handed him medicine and told him to take until it is all gone.[187]

## ERRORS CAUSED BY DRUGS RESULT IN MANY DEATHS EACH YEAR.

In between the many distractions of answering the phone, monitoring employees for theft, handing out the bathroom key, and trying to satisfy the customers who are in a hurry, pharmacists are still expected to give out a patient's prescription without errors.

Everyone makes mistakes. Since the primary role of a pharmacist is to dispense drugs, the potential for human error runs a bit higher than one might think. A good pharmacist is one who can fill those prescription bottles quickly, correctly, and sometime in a chaotic environments.

There are lots of precautionary procedures to insure that the chance for errors will be minimized. However, errors continue to occur in many aspects of healthcare.

- It is estimated that 44,000 to 98,000 patients die annually as a result of errors in patient care, along with more than 1 million patients injured annually.[188]

- Over 7000 Americans die annually from medication errors alone.[189]

- Labeling and packaging errors accounted for 33 percent of medication errors, including 30 percent of fatalities.[190]

- The United States Pharmacopeia (USP) in conjunction with the Institute for Safe Medication Practices (ISMP) maintains MEDMARX, which is an anonymous database of voluntarily reported medication errors from hospitals and health care facilities nationwide. According to reports, in 2002 more than 200,000 medication errors were documented. More than 3000 of these errors resulted in patient injury, 514 required initial or prolonged hospitalization, and 20 resulted in patient death.[191]

The number of medication errors is high, but in actuality, the numbers could be much higher. Even though all errors should be reported, that is not always the case. The scenario is somewhat of a catch-22. The more errors you report, the less competent you look. Professionals may fear retribution if reporting too many errors. Also there may be times when a patient didn't realize that an error occurred and therefore did not report it.

## ADVERSE EFFECTS FROM TAKING DRUGS CORRECTLY, AS PRESCRIBED, ALSO CAUSE HARM AND SOMETIMES DEATH TO PATIENTS.

Medication errors are not the only problem. Even when a drug is taken exactly as prescribed by the medical doctor, serious problems can still occur.

- *A Journal of the American Medical Association* article estimated that more than 700,000 patients were treated in emergency departments for adverse drug events in 2004-2005. Of these visits, one-third was attributed to allergic reactions, and another one-third was due to unintentional overdoses.[192]

**219**

- There are over 106,000 deaths per year from non-error, but adverse effects of medications. These deaths are caused by taking the medications correctly, as the doctor had prescribed.[193,194]

- Many people over age 60 take multiple medications and suffer adverse effects caused by *polypharmacy*.[195]

- These effects of polypharmacy have never been tested, as drug studies involve single drugs not combinations of drugs.

## NEW SIDE EFFECTS AND PROBLEMS ARE DISCOVERED A FEW YEARS AFTER A DRUG IS SOLD ON THE MARKET.

There are multiple cases involving drugs that made it through testing and were sold on the market, only later to find that they caused harmful, sometimes fatal, side effects.

**Phen-Fen,** used for weight loss, is an example already discussed in chapter 6. It consisted of a combination of two drugs, phentermine and fenfluramine. It was pulled from the market when this combination was found to cause pulmonary hypertension and valvular heart disease in up to 30 percent of the patients.[196]

**Vioxx** was in a class of drugs known as COX-2 inhibitors. It was an anti-inflammatory, similar to ibuprofen and naproxen, yet supposedly without causing the side effects to the stomach, including ulcer. Vioxx, created by drug company Merck, was allowed to be put on the market in 2000, despite early warning that it may cause cardiovascular problems, such as heart attacks.

In fact, Vioxx did another study excluding heart patients and still found that four times as many Vioxx patients suffered from heart attacks and cardiovascular complications than those taking naproxen. Nevertheless, Vioxx was aggressively marketed. Merck hired Bruce Jenner and Dorothy Hamill and spent $160 million for advertising. Despite all the warnings that continued to come in, Merck kept selling until 2004. By the time they finally pulled it off the market over 60,000 patients had died from taking Vioxx.[197]

**220**

**Darvocet** was a painkiller which consisted of a combination of propoxyphene and acetaminophen, and it has been on the market since 1957. In 2010 it was pulled off the market after new data showed that it can increase patient's risk of serious or fatal heart rhythm abnormalities.[198]

**Floroquinolones** are a class of antibiotics, including ciprofloxacin (Cipro), levofloxacin (Levaquin), and moxifloxacin (Avelox). Additionally, there are several other medications in this class that have been pulled off the market due to various toxicities.[199] These are used for a variety of infections from bronchitis to bladder infections. There is a growing population that has been severely harmed from these drugs which cause tendonitis and neuropathy bad enough to disable young and healthy individuals. And the worst part is that they are still on the market and commonly prescribed for conditions that have other safer alternatives, or when an antibiotic isn't really necessary. For more information please read Bruce Miller's interview at the end of the chapter.

All drugs have side effects. And whenever there's a new drug on the market, as exciting as the commercials make it look, the complete side effect profile is unknown. As more patients take the drug, more side effects and complications will eventually be revealed.

## THE MAKING OF DRUGS HAS BECOME A JOKE, FILLED WITH EXAGGERATIONS, MISREPRESENTATIONS, AND PLAIN LIES.

Drug manufacturers are so disconnected from health, and so in tune to profit. Claims are exaggerated, false claims are made, and drugs are pushed onto the market to create profits as quickly as possible.

- **Business Entrepreneurship**

  Recently, I attended a business seminar with the intent of learning tips and techniques to become a successful entrepreneur. The event was well received, with over 500 people in the room. There was a breakout session named, *Creating your Unique Selling Proposition (USP)* during which each participant was randomly partnered with another, and each

each had to create a USP for his or her own business.

I brainstormed some possible USPs, such as: *Finding better solutions for managing one's healthcare,* and *Helping people get off their meds and find alternative solutions.*

Once again, this seminar was about starting a business, and certainly not specific to the health or pharmaceutical industries. Ironically, my partner for this exercise happened to run his own business which was a laboratory that performed independent tests on new medications. His business is successful when drug companies use his laboratory to test their drugs. His USP was: *Get new medications on the market faster.*

That was a rather odd synchronicity, and yes, I was very annoyed.

- **David Franklin, Whistleblower**

David Franklin is scientist with a PhD in microbiology. His goal was to have a career in research. He applied for jobs at several pharmaceutical companies. When he couldn't land a job, he then applied for the sales representative position at Warner-Lambert as a way to get his foot in the door. He hoped to eventually transfer to a position in the research department.

During the interview process, Franklin was not questioned about his research experience, or his background. Instead, he was asked some odd questions, like "How do you feel about bending the rules?"

Franklin's first job was to work with their new drug for epilepsy, Neurontin. Neurontin's sales were slow and disappointing. The company wanted to get as many sales as possible before the patent expired and competitors would be allowed to make a generic equivalent.

Even though Neurontin was only FDA approved for epilepsy, executives had pushed Franklin to sell Neurontin to doctors and mention that it treated a variety of other conditions, such as bipolar disorder, migraines, attention deficit disorder, and sexual dysfunction.

Even though there were no studies to back up these claims, and even though the FDA did not approve of the uses, Franklin was still instructed to sell Neurontin as treatment for these other conditions. Since Franklin had a PhD and a *doctor* title before his name, he therefore had more credibility when selling. He was instructed to gain access to the neighborhood physicians by using his credentials, and then explain to those doctors that Neurontin could be used for a wide range of neurological problems.

There were many clinical trials that showed Neurontin doesn't help neurological conditions. These studies were filed away and kept hidden from public view.

In 1996 Franklin filed a whistleblower lawsuit against Warner-Lambert for using an illegal marketing plan to drive up sales. Franklin also testified that their marketing plan included paying doctors to put their names on articles written about Neurontin by ghostwriters, and paying doctors to speak at conferences about the drug.

Warner-Lambert pled guilty to two counts of violating the Food, Drug and Cosmetic Act, for misbranding Neurontin, and was ordered to pay a $430 million criminal fine. David Franklin was awarded $24 million for his whistleblowing.[200, 201, 202]

- **Clinical studies are often biased because they are created by the drug manufacturers themselves.**

  ° Most clinical trials are conducted by the pharmaceutical company that manufactures and sells the drug.

  ° When reviewing the data for antidepressants such as Zoloft, in more than half the studies the sugar pill was shown to relieve the patient's depression as well as, or better than, the Zoloft pill.[203]

○ In the late 1990s Pfizer's drug Diflucan, which is an anti-fungal, was promoted to women as the "neat treatment" for yeast infection.[204] Pfizer tested the drug against two older antifungals. However, the doctors had the patients swallow the older two drugs orally, even though it was known that neither drug would work when swallowed by mouth. One had to be taken intravenously, and the other was effective only in a cream form. In other words, Pfizer set up the trial in a way so that Diflucan would come out as the superior drug.[205]

○ According to David Franklin, "You can design an experiment to prove anything you want."[206]

With many clinical trials are rigged, and claims exaggerated or false, the making of pharmaceuticals has become a joke. Consumers can no longer believe the study results or statistics that they hear about drugs.

## THE FOOD AND DRUG ADMINISTRATION (FDA) NO LONGER HAS THE CONSUMERS GOOD HEALTH AS THEIR FIRST PRIORITY.

The Food and Drug Administration's mission is: "Protecting consumers and enhancing public health by maximizing compliance of FDA regulated products and minimizing risk associated with those products."[207]

Yet the FDA is highly influenced by the pharmaceutical companies.

**The FDA allows direct-to-consumer advertising** which allows more people to be exposed to more appealing and biased advertisements about drugs.

**FDA approved drugs are later pulled off market.** It's not rare for the FDA to allow a drug on the market and then a few years later studies show the drug causes severe side effects and deaths. Some examples already mentioned were Phen-Fen, Vioxx, and Darvocet.

**The FDA has issued several Black Box Warnings.** A black box warning appears on the package insert for prescription drugs that may cause serious or severe side effects. Studies show that the drug carries significant risk of serious or life threatening adverse effects. The FDA can require a pharmaceutical company to place a black box warning, and it is the strongest warning before the drug is pulled off the market.[208]

However, there are several drugs that have black box warnings that doctors still commonly prescribe.

- **Ciprofloxacin, (Cipro) and Levofloxacin (Levaquin)** are commonly prescribed antibiotics with an increased risk of tendonitis and tendon rupture which can disable healthy, young adults.[209]

- **Fluoxetine (Prozac), Sertraline (Zoloft), Paroxetine (Paxil), Citalopram (Celexa)** are commonly prescribed antidepressants with an increased risk of suicidal thinking and behavior in children, and young adults with major depressive disorder (MDD) and other psychiatric disorders.[210]

- **Ibuprofen (Motrin), Naproxen (Naprosyn, Aleve), Diclofenac (Voltaren)** are in the class of drugs known as nonsteroidal anti-inflammatories (NSAIDs) and are sold over-the-counter and at higher doses by prescription. This class of drugs was found to cause an increased risk of heart attack and stroke, which can be fatal.[211]

**The FDA doesn't allow non-toxic cancer therapies on the market.** On the other side, there are many non-toxic cancer regimens that the FDA has banned and taken off the market all in the name of profit. How is it possible that chemotherapy, radiation and surgery are the only cancer treatments to pass FDA guidelines?

There's the story of two-year-old Alexander who was diagnosed with brain

**225**

cancer in 1998. The parents found a doctor in Texas, Dr. Stainslaw Burzynksi, MD, PhD who used innovative and nontoxic therapies to treat brain tumors and had successfully treated a significant number of patients. The parents decided to take their son to be treated in Texas after reading about the many severe side effects of chemotherapy, including:

*Low hemoglobin, low white blood cells, low platelets, infection, need for blood transfusion, need for platelet transfusion, pain, nausea, vomiting, hair loss, skin injury, heart damage, lung damage, liver damage, kidney damage, loss of hearing, small stature, hormonal problems such as low growth hormone or low thyroid hormone, infertility, second cancer, intellectual decline, worsening of neurological symptoms, ineffectiveness, and death.*

However, even though the parents chose the non-toxic therapy for their son, and the doctor was willing to treat them, the FDA stepped in and would not allow it. They said the standard protocol was to do the chemotherapy and radiation, and if those failed then the alternatives would be allowed.

The parents reluctantly agreed. However, three months into chemotherapy their son complained of pain in his head and neck. Upon examination by MRI, thirty new tumors had appeared and Alexander passed away only days later.[212]

The FDA exists to protect the public health from risk of dangerous drugs. But in actuality, it allows harmful, useless products to be sold on the market when there are less expensive, natural solutions. Additionally, it doesn't allow these natural or non-toxic therapies to be sold on the market. The FDA, disguised as an agency to protect the public, in actuality is a *center of corruption*.

**EVEN WHEN A DRUG CAUSES HARM TO PATIENTS AND THE DRUG COMPANY MUST PAY A SETTLEMENT, THE AMOUNT THEY HAVE TO PAY HARDLY CREATES A DENT IN THEIR MASSIVE PROFITS.**

### David Franklin
Warner Lambert was fined $430 million after Franklin's whistleblowing. That may seem like a steep fine. However, Neurontin earned $10 billion

for the company, and approximately 90 percent was earned for uses the government had not approved. Although it may seem like a large fine, yet it's only three percent of the total drug sales. Therefore, it's merely a slap on the wrist, or the cost of doing business.[213]

## Bextra

Bextra, produced by Pfizer, was an anti-inflammatory drug that was in the same class of drug as Vioxx and came on the market in 2001. After many billions in revenue, a FDA warning was issued in 2004 due to increased risk of heart attack and stroke. Bextra was FDA approved for inflammation and menstrual cramps. However, Pfizer sales representatives promoted Bextra for off-label uses and at higher doses. In 2005, Pfizer was ordered to pay nearly $1.5 billion in a criminal fine, the largest fine the federal government has ever collected. However, Pfizer's sales revenue for 2010 was reported at $67.8 billion.

Once again, the fines are steep. However, to the drug companies they're more of a slap on the wrist and only a small percentage of the revenue. It would be like a drug dealer who made $2 million selling illegal drugs got caught and the courts ordered him pay $60,000 and sent him on his way. The fine would hardly serve as a deterrent to stop the crime.

## DRUG COMPANIES ARE NOT INTERESTED IN DRUGS THAT WILL CURE A CONDITION; THEY ARE INTERESTED IN LONG-TERM USE AND PROFIT.

**Drugs that Cure.** When there are simple solutions that can cure a disease, the medical industry and pharmaceutical companies lose billions of dollars. In the world of doctors and drugs, diseases and the body are complex things that the simple person cannot understand and it is best if they trust their doctor. In the natural health world, there are natural, simple and inexpensive cures for almost every condition. Looking back at the herbal remedy for Hepatitis B, compare dandelion root tea for $5, to the expensive, sophisticated, and toxic prescription drugs commonly used to treat the disease. If the masses learned about these simple natural cures, it could potentially cause financial ruin for the pharmaceutical companies.

**Me Too Drugs.** These are drugs that are structurally very similar to drugs that are already on the market, with only minor differences.[214] The pharmaceutical industry produces these medications as copycat drugs that are typically in the same class of medication, that often don't have much, if any, benefit over the drugs they are mimicking. These drugs are not new, they are made to create a profit.

- Seventy-five percent of all new drugs on the market can be considered *Me too drugs*, merely imitations, with slight alterations of existing medications.

- These copycats are not required to prove in testing to be better than the drug that is already on the market. They only have to work better than the placebo.

- In the past, the *Me too drugs* brought to market were tweaked improvements on its predecessor, working on more specific ailments or creating less side effects. However, today the main motivation is profit.

- The ideal *Me too drug*:

    ○ A slight modification of an existing drug.
    ○ FDA approval just in time for the first drug's patent to expire.
    ○ Studies show an added benefit of this drug over the previous.
    ○ A colorful marketing campaign.

There is often demand for the new drugs because consumers are well versed in the notion that *new* is better and more desirable. When the Prilosec patent expired in 2001, the drug manufacturer, Astra Zeneca, was ready with *me too drug* Nexium, which has generated over $4 billion in revenue.

Here are some examples, and the respective manufacturers:

- Prilosec (AstraZeneca) and Nexium (AstraZeneca)
- Claritin (Schering Plough) and Clarinex (Schering Plough)
- Zocor (Merck & Co.) and Lipitor (Pfizer, Inc.)

Once again, the *Me too drugs* account for most of the new drugs on the market.

**228**

This is another indicator that the manufacturers are not working to cure any disease, but only to make a profit.

## THE HEALTHCARE SYSTEM HAS BECOME AUTOMATED AND IMPERSONAL, AND DISCONNECTED FROM THE HUMAN TOUCH OF HEALING.

The people who make the drugs are too many degrees away from those who are sick. The ones who run the laboratory are under pressure to show positive results for a drug. The salespeople are under pressure to create big profits. The system has spiraled out of control. The doctors want the best care for their patients, yet they are only trained in drugs. The pharmaceutical companies want the biggest profits for their drugs. When a cheap non-toxic cancer therapy comes along, it threatens the livelihood of those who work for the drug companies as cheaper alternatives that are safe and effective have the potential to wipe out an industry. After learning of the many non-toxic cancer treatments that heal but were suppressed by the FDA, the bigger picture emerges.

But what happens when the son of a drug sales representative or an employee of the FDA becomes diagnosed with cancer. Now has the system gone too far?

There is no longer human connection in the healthcare fields. It has become an impersonal, profit-seeking venture. The businesses and corporations are prospering, yet the humans are paying the price.

**POINTS TO REMEMBER:**

- The pharmaceutical companies have made profit a priority above health.

- It is no longer safe to believe commercials or study statistics about pharmaceuticals.

- The pharmaceutical companies have gone way beyond anything ethical to create billions of dollars in sales.

- There are often simpler, holistic solutions to many conditions and diseases.

## INTERVIEW WITH VICTIM OF PHARMACEUTICALS
### BRUCE MILLER

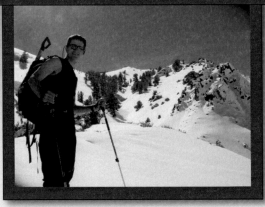

*Bruce Miller was a healthy and active man in his early thirties working as a software engineer. He took the antibiotic Cipro (ciprofloxacin) for stomach condition and soon after he developed tendonitis in his shoulder. His doctor denied that the medication could cause the health condition he was experiencing, so he continued to take it. The result was severe tendonitis to the point that he is now disabled.*

**Dr. Leyla: What was your life like before?**
Bruce: I've always been fit and active. I worked out at the gym three days a week, and also I would go on hikes where I would carry 55 to 60 pounds of gear on my back. I was involved in mountaineering classes, avalanche rescue classes, and I was preparing for a class to use an ice axe to climb in snow and mountains.

**Dr. Leyla: What kind of work did you do?**
Bruce: I was a software engineer up until I had to go on disability.

**Dr. Leyla: What drug did the doctor prescribe to you and for what condition?**
Bruce: He prescribed three courses of Cipro for small intestine bacterial overgrowth. This was caused by an area in my digestive tract that had low motility, so the food wouldn't move along as it was supposed to and it would cause some gas and bloating. I had it all my life, and my dad and grandfather also had it.

**Dr. Leyla: When did you take the medication?**
Bruce: The first time was in March of 2010.

**Dr. Leyla: When you picked up the prescription did the pharmacist counsel you about the medication?**
Bruce: No, the pharmacist was on a break and not available for consultation. When I picked it up the clerk just marked the *refuse counseling* box and asked me to sign.

**Dr. Leyla: Did you read about the side effects and warnings?**
Bruce: Yes, I saw the warnings. The side effects cause problems in a small percentage of the population. I was healthy, and I didn't have a history of having bad reactions to drugs, nor did anyone else in my family. I didn't feel that I had any reason to believe that I'd be in that minority percentage. Also I had taken Cipro a decade before and didn't have any problems.

**Dr. Leyla: When did you first start getting symptoms?**
Bruce: About a month later, although I didn't know they were from the Cipro. I was already going to a physical therapist as I had tendonitis of the external and internal rotators in my shoulder. But then I developed tendonitis in my biceps as well.

**Dr. Leyla: Did you question the doctor?**
Bruce: Yes, I went back and told him about my shoulder. He gave me a steroid, prednisone, for a back strain, but it made both my back and the tendonitis even worse. It took 10 weeks to recover.

**Dr. Leyla: How bad was it?**
Bruce: It was severe enough to limit mobility. Every time I took a step I felt pain in my shoulder. If I was riding in a car and felt a bump, it was also extremely painful. It got to the point that when I went shopping I would use the electric cart.

**Dr. Leyla: What happened next?**
Bruce: In June, I took the second prescribed course of Cipro. At this point I hadn't made the connection of the Cipro causing my problems.

**Dr. Leyla: How did your body respond?**
Bruce: After two weeks the symptoms got much worse. My shoulder got even worse as well. I couldn't walk during most of the month.

**Dr. Leyla: Was the doctor aware of the severe drug interaction of Cipro and prednisone? According to Drugs.com, "Concomitant administration of (Cipro and) corticosteroids (such as prednisone) may potentiate the risk of tendonitis and tendon rupture."[1]**

Bruce: Yes, but he told me he had given thousands of steroid shots in his career and just ignore it. Since then, I've learned that steroids cause permanent type 2 diabetes, cataracts, cartilage destruction, nerve damage, etc. in rates higher than 1 in 1000. So I can assume I'm not the only one who has been injured.

**Dr. Leyla: Did you notice the connection to taking the Cipro?**

Bruce: Yes, I read the package insert once again. There are a whole mess of side effects listed, but there is also a black box warning that Cipro may rupture tendons. I had known Levaquin, (a drug in the same class as Cipro) was dangerous to tendons for several years. When had I questioned my doctor about it the first time it was prescribed, he replied that Cipro wasn't Levaquin and in all his years he had never seen a case of tendonitis caused by the drug. I also asked my sports medicine doctor so I could have a second opinion. He didn't believe it was possible. He thought that those side effects only occurred in those older than 60, and only caused Achilles tendon problems.

**Dr. Leyla: Were you then convinced?**

Bruce: No, I then went to another sports medicine doctor. I pointed out that the package insert mentioned that you can get tendonitis in other areas of the body as well. His reply, as close as I can remember it, was "Then tear up the package insert and throw it away. Never read a package insert again. You are putting bad ideas in your head." I was shocked. To me it meant that I had these problems for some other natural reasons, I was blaming them on the drugs, and I shouldn't read the drug warnings because there was no relationship. It made me think that it was merely a coincidence that I was getting these symptoms shortly after taking the drugs, or that the symptoms were in my head.

**Dr. Leyla: So then what happened?**

Bruce: After being reassured by all three doctors that I asked, I was then scheduled for another round of Cipro, which I took in August. My condition got much worse much quicker. Within a week, I had ten different tendonitises in my shoulder, including all four tendons of the biceps muscle, which does not happen by natural causes. September 8, 2010 was my last day of work before I went on disability.

**Dr. Leyla: How has your condition progressed?**
Bruce: I continued a slow decay for the next three months. Every few days brought a new tendonitis, joint pain, or loss of joint articulation. If a tendon developed tendonitis in one side of my body, I was assured it would appear on the other side within 48 hours. I was very limited and I had to use crutches for nine months, as well as an electric mobility scooter some of the time.

**Dr. Leyla: Besides the side effects, did Cipro cure your condition?**
Bruce: No, it's a genetic condition, so it can't be cured by an antibiotic. But the doctor said that some people get cured for the rest of their lives. He promised great and amazing results.

**Dr. Leyla: What is your life like now?**
Bruce: I can't work, and I can only walk two blocks, with resting. I now have tendonitis in my hands. I can't type and it's difficult to use a mouse, but I can use speech-to-text. It's still very limited and I can't do spreadsheets or technical engineering. I sometimes have brain fog, and it's been so bad that I put something on a counter in front of me, I stay at the counter, and two minutes later it's lost and don't know where it is anymore, while it's still lying in front of me. I also have had some problems with eyes regarding focusing, loss of visual acuity, and dry eye symptoms. For many months, my toes and thumbs didn't bend. The last time I counted, I had 63 tendonitises at different times over the past 15 months, sometimes coming back two or three times.

**Dr. Leyla: What is the prognosis?**
Bruce: No one knows. From talking to people in the support groups who have also dealt with this, I believe that you eventually recover, but it takes a couple years. They say you never get back to 100 percent.

**Dr. Leyla: What are you doing to recover?**

Bruce: Lots and lots of supplements. I also go to Aquatherapy and physical therapy. Besides that, I'm waiting it out.

**Dr. Leyla: In 2010 Levaquin was the 21st top selling drug, earning $1.35 billion. Although there is a generic available for Cipro, it spent years as the top selling antibiotic.[2] Yet, Cipro and other drugs in that class have a black box warning for tendonitis. Are you planning to sue and hold the pharmaceutical companies responsible for the damage they caused?**

Bruce: After speaking with attorneys about my situation and that of many others I've met, I found out the black box warning puts the responsibility on the consumer and actually serves to protect the drug companies from being held liable. Also, I had been injected with a second drug, betamethasone, which is also known to affect the tendons. So it would be a difficulty to show Cipro as the only cause. As I understand it, it would be almost impossible for me to take them to court and win.

However, there are many others in my support group that have suffered from neuropathy, for which these antibiotics do not have a black box warning. So they may have a good case.

**Dr. Leyla: I understand that you are working to help others in this situation, or better yet, to avoid it. What are you doing to be proactive?**

Bruce: I've met 25 people in eight states who have this condition, I'm involved in online support groups, and I'm also collecting a picture book of people who have been injured by these drugs.

**Dr. Leyla: What is your goal?**

Bruce: I want to understand what happened to me, and I want to recover. It's very random, as some people who don't do anything recover faster. As an engineer, I've always worked to figure things out. Now I'm using those skills for a different purpose.

**Dr. Leyla: Have you considered alternative or natural healthcare options for your recovery?**
Bruce: Yes, I went to an acupuncturist, and I did hypnotherapy which has helped me cope with my situation. I've also participated in group meditations that were very helpful.

**Dr. Leyla: You listened to your doctor, were compliant with your medications, did your research, and read about the drug. You acted intelligently and responsibly, yet you still ended up with severe and disabling side effects. What can you, and others as well, do to prevent these situations, which in fact occur much more often than many realize?**
Bruce: Don't take any drugs. (Laughter) They're all so dangerous and I think that most people don't realize the extent of how potentially damaging they really are.

**Dr. Leyla: Do you blame the doctor or drug company more?**
Bruce: They're really both at fault. I'm disappointed with the doctors because I asked so many, and they completely disregarded what I pointed out on the package insert and my concerns. In fact, one doctor had told me that he had never seen a case of tendonitis in his years of practice. But I met a person in my support group who was disabled by the same drug and happened to go to the very same doctor a month before. So the doctor plain lied. I think he was getting ready to retire and had no desire to spend time looking into my situation.

**Dr. Leyla: How do you feel about your experience and recovery? Have you been dealing with a lot of emotions?**
Bruce: I definitely feel hopeful. I feel that I know how to handle my thoughts and that makes me much better prepared psychologically to handle this. Almost immediately, I brought my mind into a survival mode, where among other things I don't think more than two days ahead or two days in the past. Also, I don't, for example, go and watch people snowboard—then I'd think about how I used to do that. Any of that would be depressing. I can watch people do things I've never done, because that won't bring back memories and create comparisons to my current condition.

**Dr. Leyla: What will you do when you recover?**
Bruce: I'd love to go snowboarding, or go hiking again. It's been about three years. My muscles have to be rebuilt.

**Dr. Leyla: How has your perspective of life and the world changed after going through this experience?**
Bruce: It's sad that you have to learn to be your own doctor, because you can't rely on the doctors to take care of you, you can't rely on a pharmacist to help you, and you can't depend on a drug to treat your condition.

**Dr. Leyla: Some drugs come on the market and the side effects and dangers are quickly discovered and a drug is pulled off the market. Yet Cipro has been on the market for over 20 years. Why do you think more people haven't had side effects and why hasn't it been pulled off the market yet?**
Bruce: I had taken Cipro once before without any problem, and yet when I did have a problem it started over a month after taking the drug. I think there may be a lot more people out there that have been affected yet have not associated their symptoms with taking Cipro, Levaquin, or Avelox because of the delayed onset. There just aren't medical tests that reveal these kinds of damages.

Also as far as reporting side effects, there is only a voluntary reporting system called Medwatch.[3] Therefore, many times side effects may not be reported, and people may not know a drug is causing symptoms. Of course the drug companies are not going to spend any time or effort discovering side effects, and they will ignore anything that they can get away with. Doctors won't report adverse reactions because it's not mandatory and they are afraid of creating a liability. My understanding is that in France, where drug adverse reaction reporting is mandatory, drugs like Cipro, Levaquin, and Avelox are estimated to have about 21 times the problem rate as is reported in the U.S.

**Dr. Leyla: You've been active with support groups. Generally speaking, what are the similarities and differences with their experiences compared to yours?**

Bruce: Most people are worse off, and many have neuropathy. I've met 25 people who are suffering with symptoms as well, and there are over 1600 people in the online support groups. My last boss' Achilles tendon ruptured, although he has completely recovered. I've met some people who have very severe symptoms.

The most common symptoms in a classic case include bilateral tendonitis and bilateral joint pain. Any joints can be affected, but especially the knees, fingers, big toes, hips, and Achilles tendon. While taking the drug some people might also develop central nervous system (CNS) symptoms like anxiety and panic attacks, visual disturbances, hallucination, nightmares, impaired short-term memory, confusion, and headaches. The whole syndrome starts most typically while taking the drug or four to eight weeks afterwards, but it can be as delayed as nine months. Also, peripheral neuropathy is very common—most commonly affecting the legs and feet. Neuropathy can feel like electrical zaps, tingling, numbness, burning, buzzing, a sense of pressure, water running down, or bugs running under the skin. About two-thirds as many get it in their legs or in their arms, including the forearms, wrists, hands and fingers. And two-thirds of those get neuropathy of the face, head, and even teeth, which I hear is terribly excruciating. There can also be muscle pain, chronic muscle hardness, fatigue, persistent gastrointestinal problems, ringing in the ears, phantom tastes and smells, eye damage causing permanent floaters, and poor circulation to the hands and feet. Although the syndrome most commonly presents as several concurrent tendonitises, a good percentage get neuropathy and CNS symptoms. There are a few people I've met who have neuropathy without the tendonitis. Food sensitivities to things like caffine, soy, sugar, gluten, and MSG are also very common all around. Those exacerbate symptoms.

**Dr. Leyla: How has this experience changed you?**
Bruce: I've come to appreciate much smaller things that I formerly took for granted—I have to. I've lost the ability to engage in my hobbies. I take life one day at a time.

For more information on quinolone toxicity:

**SaferPills.org
Facebook.com/
FluoroquinoloneToxicity**

For stories of people affected by quinolone toxicity:

**Facebook.com/pages/The-
Fluoroquinolone-Wall-of-
Pain/209182505773463**

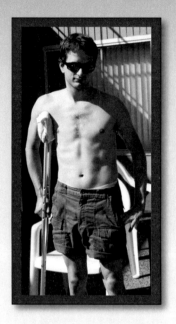

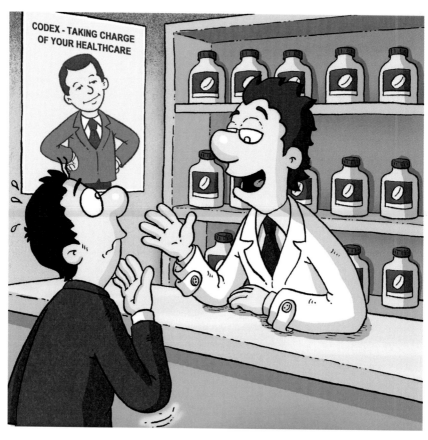

THAT'S CORRECT, ALL OUR NATURAL PRODUCTS MUST NOW BE ISOLATED, CHEMICALLY STABILIZED, SATURATED WITH PRESERVATIVES TO ENSURE SHELF LIFE, AND INJECTED WITH FLAVOR AND COLORING TO CAMOUFLAGE THE CHEMICALS AND LOOK AND SMELL FRESH.

# CHAPTER 14

# THE GAMEPLAN
## (FOR WORLD DOMINATION)

*If people let the government decide what foods they eat and what medicines they take, their bodies will soon be in as sorry a state as are the souls of those who live under the tyranny.*
*~Thomas Jefferson*

In summary, the pharmaceutical companies, in conjunction with insurance, the FDA, and the media, have created an extremely successful and powerful business system.

The methodology is relatively simple:

1. Create a drug.
2. Manage the testing of the medicine to ensure FDA clearance.
3. Carve a message via advertising that sparks emotions and thus ignites demand.
4. Watch in glee as the dollars roll in.

*Gotta have it, or I'll definitely die, or worse*—this is the stuff of successful drug marketing. American society conveys in a variety of ways, blatantly and subtly, that drugs are desirable, effective, superior, and normal.

However, the pharmaceutical companies have evolved into much more than just a profitable business for healthcare. In fact, they have slowly been working to create a very dangerous world, all in the name of profit.

So what is their gameplan?

## THE GAMEPLAN

☑ **Make People Want Drugs.** The demand is there. Prescription drugs are convenient, and give the promise of a quick fix. The average American will turn to drugs in their time of sickness.

☑ **Experts Recommend Drugs.** American society's most trusted *experts*, doctors and pharmacists, provide the stamp of approval by recommending prescription products to the masses, based on information they're fed by the drug's manufacturers. Many physicians effectively act as glorified sales reps for the drug manufacturers.

☑ **Doctors are trained only on Drugs.** Medical students learn many thousands of facts about how the body works, and how to treat illnesses with drugs and surgery. They learn very little about natural forms of treatment or the benefits of other forms of alternative healthcare. Much of the contemporary Western medical syllabus has been developed over the last half century in close association with the pharmaceutical industry. Even though patients expect doctors to be experts in healthcare, they are trained primarily in drugs.[215]

☑ **Use Drugs Instead of Prevention.** There is very limited proper training of medical doctors about the merits of nutritional and lifestyle management. Very few medical schools provide adequate training in nutrition, and even fewer receive any meaningful training on lifestyle management techniques.[216] Their education minimizes any effective efforts in the direction of disease prevention. The most profitable companies have the most advertising dollars and therefore the loudest voices. There is no profit in disease prevention; the greatest profit comes after a patient is sick.

☑ **Insurance Approves Drugs.** When a health insurance approves and pays for a drug on the health plan, this not only makes the medication affordable for the patient, but it also serves to validate and further promote the covered medications. Additionally, health insurance guidelines rarely cover non-standard or alternative forms

242

of healing or prevention, thus making them appear even less worthy or acceptable.

☑ **FDA Approves Drugs.** The Food and Drug Administration serves as regulation that determines whether or not the drug being tested is considered to be safe and effective. The public puts their trust and health in the hands of FDA's stamp of approval. However, the FDA often approves drugs that harm or kill patients, and also restricts or bans holistic practices that can help heal patients.

☑ **Drugs are in Commercials.** The pharmaceutical companies use their massive profits to advertise in all forms of media, including television, radio, internet, magazines, and newspapers, creating a normal presence.

☑ **Persuade the public there is a Pill for every Illness.** After gathering information from the media to the doctors, most people believe the most appropriate course of action when faced with a disease is to go to their physician to get a prescription drug. Patients generally don't understand that the drug prescribed may only relieve symptoms of the illness and it's unlikely that it will deal with its root cause. Additionally, patients rarely fully understand the side effects of the drugs they take.

☑ **Bad Food Means More Profit.** Food companies sell a variety of foods that the average person can't resist. They make us fat and predispose us to a higher risk of diabetes, cancer and heart disease.[217] At the same time these foods are highly convenient, inexpensive, very accessible and even addictive. The priorities of these big food companies are to gain maximum dollars and profit, and not to provide healthy, nutrient-rich food. Therefore, they fill our supermarkets with less-than-healthy, generally heavily processed foods, rich in simple carbohydrates and fats, and deficient in healthy nutrients. These foods are making us sick at an unprecedented rate.[218]

☑ **The Sicker the Better.** Increase the rates of chronic disease among the public so pharmaceutical companies can expand their market.

**243**

There is little incentive for pharmaceutical interests, or healthcare providers whose livelihoods or profits are based on sales of pharmaceuticals, to prevent sickness. This sets the scene perfectly for the pharmaceutical companies to come in with its medicine chest of profitable drugs. *The earlier people start getting sick and the longer they live, the bigger the market.* Chronic disease incidence is increasing in younger and younger age groups. Additionally, the average life spans are beginning to shorten primarily because of the effects of obesity.[219]

☑ **Only Drugs and Chemotherapy approved for Cancer.** The standard Western Medicine treatment for cancer is chemotherapy, radiation, and surgery. Doctors are not trained in any other form of cancer treatment. In addition, it is illegal for doctors to recommend other non-toxic forms of cancer treatment.[220]

☑ **Discredit Alternative Medicine as *Quacks*.** Medical doctors, who are the recognized experts of health, are trained to considered alternative forms of healthcare as inferior. Additionally, the FDA does not recognize the benefits of most alternative forms of healthcare. Therefore, the general belief is these other alternative forms of health care are considered inferior, untrustworthy and untested—said to be promoted only by quacks and those *new-age folks.*

☑ **Create Laws to Increase Pharmaceutical Company's Profits.** With their massive profits, the pharmaceutical industry has lobbied to create rules, regulations and laws that will benefit their business. One example is in the 1990s the pharmaceutical companies lobbyied so they could advertise their drugs directly to consumers, which increased demand of their drugs and their profits.[221]

☐ **Create Regulation to push natural products and Supplements off the Market.** The next goal of the gameplan is to make natural products unavailable to the public. There are laws being developed and implemented in the US, Canada, the European Union (EU), Australia and other countries that aim to create rules and regulations that would be impossible for natural product manufacturers to

**244**

comply with.[222]   In essence, they are working to tighten the regulatory noose around natural health companies as these laws make it progressively harder to market effective natural products that, in many cases, are able to completely replace the need for drugs if used in conjunction with healthy diets and lifestyles.

Regulators often claim that the laws they are developing to regulate natural products are aimed at protecting consumers.  Yet, natural products are the safest things we routinely place in our mouths, on average being around one thousand times safer than the average food, and around one hundred thousand times safer than the average drug.[223]  These rules are about setting an obstacle course that is impassable by smaller companies.

They are trying to regulate:

- Types of products available, including their dosage.
- Claims that can be used that help inform a potential consumer of its benefits to their health.

The smaller companies have long been the pioneers and innovators in the natural products industry.

The lawmakers are claiming that this is necessary for consumer safety.  However, this is in itself absurd given that drugs are the most dangerous substances typically ingested by humans.[224]  If this does pass, many natural products that can prevent disease will be unavailable for purchase.

☐ **Prohibit Alternative Healthcare Options.**  The only Option Left will be Doctors and Drugs.

If these regulations come into effect, many herbals and natural products used by the classic alternative healthcare providers, such as Ayruvedic Medicine and Traditional Chinese Medicine will no longer be able to practice as they have been doing for the past few thousand years.  This is a step towards the elimination of the many forms of alternative healthcare.

## THE NEW WORLD OF PHARMACEUTICAL MONOPOLY

If their gameplan is successful, the new world will have doctors and drugs as the only healthcare option. The bountiful world of alternative healthcare will be a practice of the past. As most people now rely on doctors and drugs, most aren't aware of the danger and therefore aren't ready to fight the battle.

## WHAT YOU CAN DO—WHAT WE MUST DO—WHICH OF THESE WILL YOU COMMIT TO?

- Stop relying on doctors and drugs for your healthcare needs.

- Take responsibility for your own health and find out how you can optimize your diet and lifestyle so that you minimize your risk of disease and enjoy the highest level of health and wellbeing possible.

- Find holistic health practitioners in your area. You can contact integrative medical associations like the International College of Integrative Medicine (www.icimed.com) to find a qualified integrative medicine practitioner in your area.

- Opt out of buying all your foods from the large supermarkets, and especially those foods that are heavily processed or that contain artificial preservatives colors or flavors. How you use your wallet is one of the most powerful tools you have!

- Avoid buying any genetically engineered foods or genetically modified organism (GMO); see the Institute for Responsible Technology's 'Non-GMO Shopping Guide' (www.responsibletechnology.org/docs/Non-GMO-Shopping-Guide.pdf).

- Consume unprocessed whole foods, a diverse range of fruits and vegetables (eat a rainbow every day!) and minimize your consumption of simple carbs and trans fats.

- Do all you can to help combat unfair regulatory restrictions on natural

**246**

health. Follow and support the work of the Alliance for Natural Health (www.anhinternational.org). They are doing amazing work that is funded only by donations in both the USA (www.anh-usa. org) and Europe (www.anh-europe.org). Both organizations work closely together in their respective territories issue regular calls to action that you will receive if you sign up for their free online newsletters. Some of the worst manifestations of these regulatory regimes are being developed by European authorities, so it's in the interests of Americans to do all we can to knock them out at source. Sitting on the sidelines is simply not an option if you care about your—and the next generation's—future and want to manage your health naturally.

## POINTS TO REMEMBER:

- The pharmaceutical companies have made profit a priority at the expense of health.

- You cannot rely upon regulatory agencies, doctors, or pharmaceutical drugs for good health.

- Alternative Healthcare Options are the best options for many health conditions.

- Regulatory agencies are working to eliminate alternative and holistic healthcare options.

## INTERVIEW WITH ALLIANCE FOR NATURAL HEALTH FOUNDER DR. ROBERT VERKERK

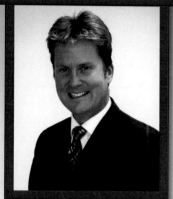

*Robert Verkerk PhD is the founder as well as executive and scientific director of the Alliance for Natural Health International (ANH-Intl). He is an internationally acclaimed scientist, with 30 years of academic, commercial and campaign experience in sustainability as it relates to the environment, agriculture and health.*

*The ANH-Intl is an internationally-active, nonprofit, non-governmental organization, based in the United Kingdom, that is working to develop more sustainable, natural and biologically-compatible approaches to healthcare.*

*As an alliance, the ANH-Intl brings together—globally—consumers, scientists, medical doctors, integrative practitioners, lawyers and other interested persons—all with a common interest to protect and promote natural health.*

**Dr. Leyla: What motivated you to start the Alliance for Natural Health back in 2002?**
Dr. Verkerk: Natural products, be they herbs from long-standing eastern or other traditional medicinal cultures or sophisticated food supplements and functional foods, continue to help millions of people to maintain or restore balance in their bodies, so that self-healing processes are able to function optimally and good health is maintained or resumed.

But therapeutic natural products are now deeply under threat, in Europe especially but also internationally, as increasingly stringent regulatory requirements are being ushered in by pharmaceutically-biased regulators, supported by a clutch of transnational corporations in the pharmaceutical and food sectors.

248

**Dr. Leyla: What do you mean by "therapeutic natural products are deeply under threat?"**

Dr. Verkerk: In many countries, including across the 27 Member States of the European Union (EU), but also in the USA, food supplements are presently classified as a category of food. This means that they are distinct from medicines (drugs), which, by definition, are products used to treat, prevent or cure disease. The European definition of a drug goes one step further by making any product that has significant pharmacological (drug-like), immunological or metabolic effects a drug.

This effectively gives drug regulators arbitrary power to classify any beneficial food product as a drug. Drugs, unlike foods, can only go on sale after they have successfully gone through extensive evaluation of their efficacy and risks to human health. European legislators have made it increasingly clear that they want to see a distinct borderline between foods and medicines, with anything that is regarded as being *therapeutic* pushed into the medicines category.

This means that a high dose supplement or any other natural health product that is intended to have profound, positive effects on human health is increasingly at risk of being classified as a drug. It will come as no surprise that the vast majority of supplement manufacturers lack the financial muscle required to run their products through a drugs licensing regime.

**Dr. Leyla: You explained that the therapeutic natural products are deeply under threat of becoming banned from the market. How close is this to becoming a reality?**

Dr. Verkerk: In Europe, we have already seen traditional herbal medicine products, such as those used in the ancient cultures of Ayurveda and Traditional Chinese Medicine being pushed into their own drugs regime. A specific subset of European drugs laws has been developed to supposedly accommodate *traditional herbal medicinal products*. At issue here is these laws are subject to pharmaceutical standards that have been developed for conventional, largely synthetic drugs based on single or very limited combinations of active ingredients.

In short, we're finding that the vast majority of herbal products from these long-standing traditions cannot conform to the requirements that were designed specifically for them! A great deal of products associated with these great traditions are now, in Europe, effectively falling between the two stools of food and medicinal law—a kind of no-man's land that bans products by default, simply because they get pushed out of the food regime and cannot access the medicines one.

The problem stems from the fact that a new, thoroughly inappropriate regulatory system has been built around healthcare traditions that are over 4,000 years old. It simply doesn't work—and that's why the main beneficiaries of this new *traditional medicines* framework are highly concentrated and extracted herbal active constituents stabilized, typically, in a pharmaceutical matrix made of synthetic polymers and preservatives. It's akin to trying to put a square peg in a round hole. The catastrophic effect of this new regime on long-standing herbal traditions is currently forming the basis of a case that we are preparing to bring to the High Court in the UK, with the aim of getting a reference to the European Court of Justice in Luxembourg. Interestingly, there's a good deal of European case law that suggests that what European regulators have done might well be illegal.

Aside from herbs, we've already seen glucosamine, the most common natural product used for those suffering arthritic complaints, being classified as a drug in Sweden and Denmark, and the European Commission is planning, within the coming 12 months, to introduce a new law that harmonizes maximum levels of vitamins and minerals in food supplements EU-wide. No surprises that the levels being considered are non-therapeutic and well below those that might be used to help people to recover from illness.

**Dr. Leyla: So the European Food Supplements Directive goes into effect, what will natural product manufacturers need to do to keep their products on the market?**
Dr. Verkerk: The Directive has already come into effect, as of 2005. However, it is a framework directive meaning that it has different provisions,

which are brought into effect at different times. For example, a key date was the 31st of December 2009, which was the last date by which derogated forms of vitamins and minerals—those that were already on sale before the Directive came into force—could be sold if the European Food Safety Authority hadn't successfully evaluated them. So to stay on the market, manufacturers have had to submit detailed dossiers demonstrating both safety and bioavailability of the nutrient forms they want to use, if they are not already approved. This is by no means an easy job, and it's also expensive, so few additional vitamin and mineral forms have been added, and many have been lost. What this kind of *positive list* system fundamentally does is move Europe towards a pre-market authorization system for food supplements, something that has more in common with a drugs regime than a food regime. European manufacturers selling herbal products that are eligible under the fast-track drugs licensing system for *traditional herbal medicinal products*, have also been very busy trying to prepare applications for product licenses. Many are finding they simply can't meet the pharmaceutical requirements, not only because of the costs involved, but also because in the case of polyherbal products—that are typical of ancient traditional medicinal cultures—it's technically impossible to do so.

**Dr. Leyla: But isn't the European Food Supplements Directive only aiming to ensure that vitamins, herbs and other food supplements on the market are safe and that labeling provides consumers with important safety information and reflects what is actually present within the bottle? Isn't this a good thing?**
Dr. Verkerk: The two primary purposes of the Directive are:

a) To harmonize laws on food supplements so as to make it easier to sell products into and between all 27 EU Member States.
b) To provide a high level of consumer protection.

While there is no doubt that the laws require set standards for quality control, this has never been a serious problem in the EU market. The problem with harmonizing across a large trading bloc like the EU is that harmonization tends to occur in the direction of the lowest common denominator, owing to the influence of the precautionary principle which is written into general food law in the EU. This means that countries like Germany and Denmark, which have historically had very restrictive national laws on food supplements, get to have a disproportionate influence. Since the laws on supplements in Europe completely ignore benefits, European regulators are quite happy to restrict levels to the point that they prevent the nearly 500 million strong population of Europe from obtaining micronutrient levels that will support optimum health.

As far as labeling is concerned, the EU's Nutrition and Health Claims Regulation is in the process of bringing in a pre-market authorization system for health claims. This means, you can only make a health claim—a claim about a product or ingredient's specific health benefit—if it has been pre-approved by the highest food authority in Europe, the European Food Safety Authority (EFSA). Again, EFSA use very stringent criteria for demonstrating a cause and effect relationship, meaning huge numbers of claims will no longer be allowed. With so many claims removed, rather than assisting consumers, we are concerned that consumers might find it even harder to differentiate between healthy and less healthy foods.

**Dr. Leyla: If the European Food Supplements Directive is able to effectively ban natural products from the marketplace, what do you see as the short and long term consequences?**
Dr. Verkerk: The restriction of the use of food/dietary supplements and traditional herbal remedies, combined with attempts of the orthodox medical establishment to quash evidence of the benefits of complementary and alternative therapies. The continuing evolution, adoption and indeed even survival of some of the great traditional medicinal cultures, such as Ayurveda, Unani and Traditional Chinese Medicine are now threatened. In addition, orthomolecular medicine and nutritional therapy, two branches of healthcare that are reliant on the use of high dosages of vitamins and minerals are also threatened unless significant changes are made to the existing laws or legislative proposals. Of course, the desire by some to use natural means of healthcare

is such that even with regulatory bans, usage will continue with products being purchased on black or grey markets. But pushing natural healthcare underground would put a major obstacle in the way of allowing such approaches to achieve their rightful place in the mainstream of healthcare.

I personally continue to be optimistic in the long-term, although feel in the short-term things will get worse before they get better. I believe that, ultimately, a natural equilibrium will be achieved between ourselves and those parts of the environment with which we have co-evolved over millennia. Our present reliance on new-to-nature drugs will, I suspect, one day be seen as a foray that was only got to be so widely accepted because of our inadequate understanding of the subtlety of interactions between our physical, genomic and bioenergetic selves and the world around us.

**Dr. Robert Verkerk**
**Alliance for Natural Health International**
**The Atrium, Curtis Road**
**Dorking, Surrey RH4 1XA**
**United Kingdom**

**Tel: +44 (0) 1306 646600**
**Fax: +44 (0) 1306 646552**
**www.anh-europe.org (European campaign)**
**www.anh-usa.org (USA campaign)**
**www.anhinternational.org (International)**

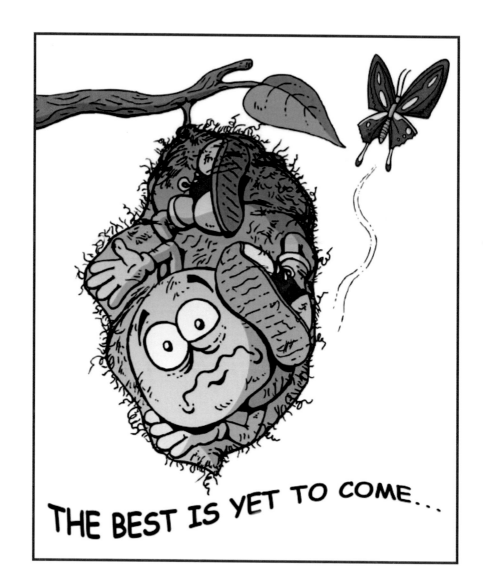

THE BEST IS YET TO COME...

# CHAPTER 15

# STARTING YOUR
# HOLISTIC JOURNEY

*Just when the caterpillar thought the world was over, it became a butterfly!*                                                    *~proverb*

If the previous chapters were successful, you've lost some faith in the medical system, and may be wondering: *So now what do I do?*

I started out with a thorough yet untested belief in doctors and drugs. It wasn't until a few years after completing pharmacy school that I came to realize the falsity of this system and started looking for new solutions. Many others seek alternative solutions only after the medical system has failed them and they have suffered with a health condition for years. Still there are others that intuitively understand completely how far astray the system has gone.

From my own research, I've learned there are many ways to heal. People have more potential to fully heal than they are led to believe. But they will never learn to tap into their own healing potential by going to a medical doctor.

The path to better health starts with research, choice, and awareness of the many alternative types of healthcare that are available. Huge volumes of information all profess to have the best solution for improving one's life.

*How do you begin, where do you go, and with whom do you now place your trust?*

There is no single answer to these questions. I've dipped my toes in many healing modalities of the physical, emotional and spiritual realm. Through these I have discovered there are myriad ways to heal the whole person, and everyone's journey is unique.

This chapter will provide a starter kit, based on some of my own research, as a first step to learning about alternative health care options, and starting your holistic journey.

## STARTING YOUR HOLISTIC JOURNEY

As your pharmacist, though, here is a crucial first-step suggestion:

***Don't stop taking your medications without first talking to your doctor.***
We've seen and heard this warning many times, and this is one with which
I completely agree. If you are currently on
any form of medication, your mind and
body may have developed a dependence
on these drugs (here's a reminder of the
final *balance scale* from Chapter 4).

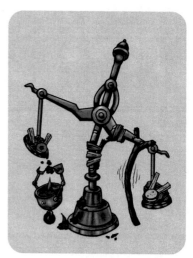

Imagine if you were severely off balance
and you removed the braces, your balance
scale would collapse. *Do not abruptly stop
taking your medication!* Instead, find an
alternative healthcare provider that can
work with your medical doctor to create
a plan to work towards that goal. Many
drugs need to be tapered down slowly so
balance can be gently restored.

**Don't rely on drugs and doctors to regain your health.** Doctors can identify problems while drugs work to alleviate symptoms. Medical doctors have excellent resources for diagnostics, and are great when you have an accident or medical emergency and need immediate care or surgery. However, their training is limited to drugs and surgery. It is important to recognize where you can benefit from doctors and drugs, where they have

**256**

limitations, and which conditions are better treated by other types of health care practitioners. Do not depend upon medical doctors for your complete health of the body, mind and spirit.

**Take responsibility.** Our society has been brainwashed to hand over control of our health to the so called *experts* in the field. Good patients are those who are *compliant* and listen to their doctors and pharmacists. Yet the person who understands your health and your body best is *you*, and it's time to take the power back. Following directions of the medical doctor is no longer the best option or the only option. You must decide that no one else is in control of your health and wellness. You must do the research, make the decisions, and take the steps towards your best health.

**Create Positive Thoughts.** Your daily thoughts create your reality, and therefore these thoughts can affect your health. Daily affirmations, as well as making a concerted effort to eliminate or minimize negative thinking, can improve health. Some thought patterns are so habitual and ingrained within us that we don't recognize them as places for improvement.

Here are examples of common thoughts (and words) people often don't realize are harmful to their health:

"I can't seem to kick this cold."

"I'm getting old."

"My body is falling apart."

"I get a terrible flu every year."

"My condition is incurable."

These statements are merely thoughts that have developed into beliefs and thus become expectations.

I was once shopping when I overheard the lady working at the check stand complaining, "I can't kick this cold." The man she was assisting replied, "You're probably beyond the worst part; it'll be gone in a day or so." I saw her eyes light up as if a new and fresh possibility had settled in. A simple shift in perspective can lighten up a person's attitude, thoughts, and reality. When the individual takes responsibility for their own attitude management, the results can be astounding.

**Create Empowering Beliefs.** Beliefs are thoughts that we accept as truth. Many patients of standard medical practice hold preconceived notions about which diseases are curable, and which are not. This only promotes failure, as often people hear a diagnosis, such as cancer, from a doctor and immediately their health worsens.

Doctors are our trusted authority on health. When doctors offer a diagnosis and tell the patient what to expect, the patient very often believes them. Yet doctors have no business considering any ailment *incurable* as they are not trained in what's possible in health in healing. Doctors are only trained in drugs and surgery, and are taught to discredit alternative therapies. For every doctor that has diagnosed a medical illness as incurable, there are patients who have regained their health through alternative means by taking back control of their own health.

In the world of alternative and holistic health, there is potential for everyone to heal. We must shift our beliefs towards anything is possible when it comes to healing.

**Meditate.** Every day our minds get filled with noise and we are inundated with useless and toxic information and images that don't serve us. Meditation has proven therapeutic significance for quieting the mind, and allowing for peaceful, uplifting thoughts. Developing a consistent meditation practice can help along the path to healing. With the advent of yoga nationwide, the acceptance level for meditation is growing exponentially.

**Dealing with Emotions.** There has been limitless research done on the impact emotions have on our wellbeing, and therefore, our health. Emotions are indicators of your state of being. Many people fear their emotions and work to suppress them, which can eventually lead to disease. There are healthy ways and techniques to deal with emotions. Most important is to not be afraid to feel the emotion. First invite it in completely, and then allow yourself to feel it, and then release it. With Somatic

**258**

Trauma Resolution, patients learn to become aware of their physical sensations as they experience an emotion. For those stuck in an emotion of anger or depression, stay connected to Abraham Hicks and the emotional scale,[225] which teaches how to always reach for a thought that feels better.[226]

**Forgive.** Forgive everyone and everything, including yourself. Forgiveness is possibly the most beneficial human attribute and is also the most ignored, or underutilized in relationships. Harboring negative emotions, no matter how justified, is clearly detrimental to the mind, body and spirit. It affects mostly the one who refuses to forgive. When we hold on to resentment or anger towards a person, that person is often unaffected and has moved on with their lives. Yet those feelings of resentment become our own problem, as we wear them in the form of health conditions and diseases. Set an intention to forgive. Sometimes just saying "I want to forgive this person" can be a difficult first step. It takes commitment, willingness and practice to forgive.[227]

**Meaning behind conditions.** Often the attitudes that come with an illness are fear and sadness. Instead of considering yourself sick, or diseased, what if you considered the situation a *health opportunity* to be thankful for? The illness forces you to come out of your daily routine and reach for a wellness state of being that you would otherwise not be inspired to achieve. It also entails seeking the positive that came out of experiencing the illness. It may sound like a stretch on day one, but it can help you feel grateful for the the journey of learning about health and well-being that your life forced you to make. Also, this possibly leads to questions, like:

What do I need to learn about this illness and myself in order to heal?

What situation or feeling am I ignoring?

What or who do I need to let go of?

Whom do I need to forgive?

What good has come out of this health condition?

Each stage is an opportunity. The miracle of the human body is that it tells you everything you need to know. By addressing underlying causes—rather than trying suppress a symptom or kill them with chemicals—a person can strive to heal and regain balance.

**Cleanse and detoxify.** There are ways to cleanse the body that range from raw food diets to colonics. Get the toxins and negative emotions out, and replace them with nutrients and healthy thoughts.

Suggested reading: Richard Anderson's *Cleanse and Purify Thyself*[228]

Suggested research: *Optimum Health Institute, Lemon Grove, Ca*


## CHOOSING A HOLISTIC PRACTITIONER

There are so many types to choose from. Do you need an acupuncturist? Or would energy work be more beneficial? What about herbals remedies? How do you know which is right for you?

**Trust your own guidance system.** Trust your instincts and intuition. Learn to rely on inner guidance to point you in the right direction and align you with those who will be beneficial. Notice if the thought of working with a certain practitioner gives you a knot in your stomach and creates tension or uneasiness. Instead, you should feel a sense of relief and lightness. Learn how to listen to your body and allow your intuition to help guide you. That's your higher-self working to lead you in the right direction.

**The Seven Planes**[229] Before knowledge about the seven planes, there was just a multitude of alternative healthcare options without much rhyme or reason. Vianna Stibal, founder of the healing technique Theta Healing, envisioned a powerful metaphysical model, where the entire universe is made up of seven dimensions all working in unison. There are healing modalities within each. Here is a summary:

> **First Plane** is made up of rocks, crystals and minerals. Crystals are a common and powerful healing modality, and minerals are necessary

for bones and good health.

**Second Plane** is where plants, herbs and nature collide; the sacred interaction between earth/air/light from which many healing modalities emanate. This is the source of homeopathy and herbalism.

**Third Plane** is the plane of the animal world, connected to motion and movement. Humans are most connected to this plane. Healing modalities would include nutrition, massage, yoga, and physical therapy. Western medicine is also in this plane as it involves changing the body with drugs and surgery.

**Fourth Plane** is the plane of the spirits. This is where our ancestors reside, and where we go between lifetimes. We all have a strong connection to the Fourth plane. Modalities include Native American and Polynesian healing methods, Shamanism, and psychic readings.

**Fifth Plane** also known as the *Astral Plane*, is the place of duality and polarity. Here reside good and evil, right path and wrong path. An example of fifth plane healing modality is angel readings where you contact your guardian angels for guidance.

**Sixth Plane** is the home of the Laws of the Universe, including the Law of Attraction, Law of Gravity, and Law of Time. Healing modalities include Astrology, Numerology, Sacred Geometry, and vibration machines, as well as sound and light therapies.

**Seventh Plane** is Everything, the All That Is, Ever Was, and Ever Will Be. Theta Healing is a prime example of healing from this dimension. Straight to the creator, instant healings are part of this plane.

**Research, Research, Research.** Read, ask, research and then research some more. Just as there are numerous ailments of the physical, emotional and spiritual; humanity has discovered an abundance of solutions from which to choose. Once a person decides to make the life-change towards holistic health, the next step is research. Seek guidance from those that have gone before you, and trust your heart on which methodology is best.

**Surrender.** Surrender is a realization that the healing comes from a power outside us, it is the willingness to stop trying to control the circumstances, and to find out what you need to learn and then let go. Often people in our society are taught to be action-oriented, as they must always *do* something. The action is important, but by itself it may not be enough.

**Don't buy snake oil.** This is an issue that I feel needs lots of work as there are an overwhelming amount of products available and it's difficult to know which are safe and effective. Like the pharmaceutical advertisements on the television, the products that have the biggest hype aren't necessarily the best products. It's important to do thorough research on the products available.

**Take Action.** The people who are able to heal are those who take their health in their own hands and take action through learning, research, and movement. There must be a willingness to do whatever is necessary to heal. Be willing to address issues on the mind, body and spirit level. If something doesn't work, then you're closer to finding what will—so keep going.

## SUMMARY

The journey to healing is unique for each person. As I watch people on their journeys with health opportunities, I wonder why one person is successful, while someone else is not, and why one person is able to heal, where another cannot. One thing is certain is that relying on your medical doctor will not get you there.

For this book I interviewed nine people who healed themselves. Each took a different path to regain his or her health. They may not know exactly what caused the problem, but they know something caused them to be off balance. They understood that to regain their health they must address the mind, body and spiritual aspects of their condition. There's a fire and a strong desire to heal, live, and the willingness to do whatever it takes.

I've also met some people who have tried several types of healing modalities and still have not recovered. What are they missing that they haven't been able to heal? Do they believe they can heal? Do they believe that they deserve to heal? Have they surrendered? Perhaps they haven't yet learned what the illness is trying to teach them. It's hard to know in every situation, but depending on the patient, sometimes the answer isn't *doing* something, but a shift at the spiritual level, or in the person's beliefs and being.

Unfortunately we live in a time when many of the alternative healthcare options are not covered by insurance. Even though they may save the insurance companies thousands of dollars by healing patients, still they are often not recognized as legitimate. It can be hard for patients to comprehend why they would pay $100 to $200 for a service when they can get a doctor's visit and a drug for $10. This is another point in the healthcare system where an effort needs to be made to fight against the bias towards Western medicine.

But healing does not have to be expensive. Looking back to the individuals who I interviewed, Susan Moss (chapter 10) took cancer into her own hands and healed herself with minimal costs. Dennis Kinnane's (chapter 4) customer took an herbal tea for a few dollars to treat his hepatitis B. Frank Tortorici (chapter 11) dealt with his Tourette's by using a raw food, vegan diet and training his mind and body. Storm Cole (chapter 5) knew she should start seeking alternative healthcare options when her doctor laughed at her self-diagnosis of chronic fatigue. Duncan Tooley's (chapter 8) condition was costing his insurance company $20,000 a month for treatment when he cured it with hypnotherapy. Art San (chapter 7) and Peter Bedard (chapter 15) refused drugs and surgery for their chronic *incurable* pain and both were able to find ways to heal. Frank Ferrante (chapter 12) listened to his doctors until he got the point where he ended up taking a handful of medications daily, but still felt terrible. He realized something needed to change.

As Frank Ferrante (chapter 12) from the movie *May I Be Frank*[230] once said, "When you are ready and open to heal, you'll be amazed at the people who show up to help you."

**POINTS TO REMEMBER:**

- There are many ways to heal.

- The path to health and wellness is a journey which entails growth and self-discovery of the mind, body and spirit.

## INTERVIEW WITH PETER BEDARD
### from CreateYourHealth.com

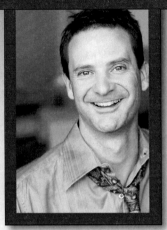

*Peter Bedard is a hypnotherapist, online producer, and actor who lives in Los Angeles, California. Peter was a young aspiring actor and dancer when he got into a moped accident which led to his suffering with back pain for 15 years. Doctors recommended surgery but he declined, as he had witnessed the pain and struggling that his father faced after his vertebrae had been fused together. Peter discovered acupuncture through a friend's referral. Unable to walk, he literally crawled into his first appointment, yet was able to walk out the office door.*

**Dr. Leyla: What was your life like before your health challenges?**
Peter: As a teenager, I was a singer, dancer, and actor. I did improvisation groups. I was energetic and I was headed for a bright future in entertainment.

**Dr. Leyla: How did that change?**
Peter: When I was 17, I was riding my moped late at night coming home from a show. Someone in a car started playing chicken with me and ran me off the road. I crashed into the back of a semi-trailer truck. I split my wrist open, my left leg and knee were shattered, and I cracked several vertebrae.

**Dr. Leyla: How was the recovery?**
Peter: The bones in my left leg were shattered into little pieces—it was in a full cast for several months with a long screw through the entire joint. I also had a full cast on my right arm. The back issues were not actually discovered until years later. I had constant pain in my back and knee from this point, up until just a few years ago.

**Dr. Leyla: What other kinds of health conditions did you suffer with?**

Peter: The accident caused pain that led to several other problems—depression, anxiety, asthma, allergies, and arthritis. I was also diagnosed with fibromyalgia. Being in constant pain created a cascade effect. One leg was longer than the other, so my spine was off kilter and I was leaning to one side. I had no cartilage in my left knee, so there was bone rubbing on bone. In my twenties, I also had sciatica, due to the damaged vertebrae and my body being out of alignment. When I was about 26 years old, I reached a point where the pain was so severe that I couldn't get out of bed for nearly two weeks.

**Dr. Leyla: How did you finally relieve that pain?**

Peter: A friend told me about an acupuncturist. He saw that I was in a lot of pain and told me about an acupuncturist. He said he had heard about this guy and I needed to go see him. So I went. I couldn't walk. I actually had to lie on my back and crawl like a crab, as it hurt too much to walk or crawl normally. In this fashion, I somehow made it to my car, drove to his office and up a flight of stairs. I probably looked ridiculous, but it was the only way I could move. After the session I was able to stand up and walk out of his office almost pain-free. This was amazing to me.

**Dr. Leyla: Did you continue to see him?**

Peter: Yes, I kept seeing him as he continued to help with my knee pain. He also recommended some Chinese herbs that helped with the pain, my digestion, and all sorts of other things.

**Dr. Leyla: Were you then on the path to recovery?**

Peter: Well, not exactly. There were lots of other things that needed to be healed. In my mid-thirties I had another problem with my back. After two weeks of unbearable pain, I once again had to try something new, as my original acupuncturist had passed on. This time I went to a chiropractor who was also referred by a friend. He was phenomenal, in that he found my sciatica was not the cause. Rather the source of the pain came from my Psoas muscle—a long, thin abdominal muscle that runs from the front to the back of the body. He applied pressure and release to it, and this action provided the relief I so desperately sought. Muscles learn to move within a particular pattern, and after the accident, my muscles were off. I had to relearn how to use my abdominal muscles properly.

Additionally, I recently healed my knee pain with Prolotherapy. Now I can finally walk without knee pain.

**Dr. Leyla: Can you explain how Prolotherapy works?**
Peter: In the Prolotherapy procedure the doctor injected dextrose, or sugar, into my knee, and through the inflammatory process I was able to build back cartilage. It helped with the bone-on-bone pain that I had been suffering with for years! It takes the place of knee replacement surgery with results that are amazing!

**Dr. Leyla: What kind of prognosis did the medical doctors offer?**
Peter: Basically, the doctors wanted me to not move and to stay in bed 24/7. But I had to go to work; I had bills to pay. They wanted me to consider surgery, and gave me all kinds of drugs and muscle relaxants, which I hated. My dad broke his back when he was nineteen, and the doctors fused it together. He has been in pain ever since. Not only did he never find adequate pain relief, but also I watched as the dose of his medications became stronger and stronger. So, in my mind, surgery was not an option.

**Dr. Leyla: How is your health and life today?**
Peter: Great. I'm pain free. I feel like a normal person, although right now I'm dealing with low testosterone levels. I tried all types of alternatives—energy work, homeopathy, naturopathy, Reiki, exercise, nutrition and supplements—but nothing helped. Now I'm on hormones, a form of conventional medicine. My energy is back, and I don't feel weak, sad or depressed. It's amazing! I'm a big believer of having choices and using whatever combination works, where you're in charge—not listening to a dictating doctor—but a health provider that is part of your personal team. I believe in integrative healing, which can

267

be alternative, conventional, or a combination of both working together.

**Dr. Leyla: You've struggled through a long, painful journey to regain your health. What advice would you give someone who is struggling with a health challenge?**
Peter: First step is to take responsibility for who you are and where you are. You have to stop blaming people and pointing the finger at those who did you wrong—life, friends, family, abusers, whatever. You have to stop looking for people to heal you and start looking for people to partner WITH you so you can heal yourself. Then it's about research and finding things that will benefit you. Healing is a process, a combination of actions and attitudes. It has to be done through the body, mind, and spirit.

**Dr. Leyla: Looking back, what could you have done differently to spare yourself all those years of suffering?**
Peter: I wish I had known about alternative medicine early on and had been around people who supported it. I wish I had found Prolotherapy right after my accident. Instead, I spent 15 to 20 years trying to find my voice. Dance was how I learned to express myself and how I communicated. When I was no longer able to dance, my voice was taken and I wasn't able to communicate or have fun.

**Dr. Leyla: Please tell us about your mission and website.**
Peter: My mission is to empower people with choices for healing and help them create vibrant health through my website, **CreateYourHealth. com.** I have a collection of fifty 5-minute introductory videos that I have created with a variety of alternative healthcare practitioners. This provides an information database for those seeking to learn about alternative and holistic health care options. My mission is to provide healing across the planet.

**Peter Bedard**
**CreateYourHealth.com**

# ENDNOTES

## INTRODUCTION

1 kff.velir.com/rxdrugs/upload/Effects-of-Direct-to-Consumer-Advertising-on-Medication-Choice-the-Case-of-Antidepressants.pdf

2 usgovinfo.about.com/od/healthcare/a/usmedicated.htm

3 www.biopsychiatry.com/medication.html

4 ezinearticles.com/?History-of-Alternative-Medicine&id=275778

5 educate-yourself.org/fc/

6 acswebcontent.acs.org/landmarks/landmarks/penicillin/penicillin.html

7 www.nytimes.com/2012/04/22/magazine/the-science-and-history-of-treating-depression.html?pagewanted=all&_r=0

8 www.nytimes.com/2011/06/05/fashion/viagra-the-thrill-that-was-cultural-studies.html?pagewanted=all

9 www.thalidomide.ca/history-of-thalidomide/

10 www.thenaturalguide.com/natural-medicine-suppression.htm

## CHAPTER 1

11 Kiyosaki, Robert T. *Rich Dad, Poor Dad.* New York, New York: Warner Books, 1998

12 Anderson, Richard, ND. *Cleanse and Purify Thyself.* Medford, Oregon: Christobe Publishing, 1988

13 DiPiro, JT, Talbert, RL. *Pharmacotherapy, A Pathophysiologic Approach.* Stanford, CT: Appleton & Lange, 1997

## CHAPTER 2

14 www.sageherbalhealing.com/herbalmedicine.html

15 www.tcmcentral.com/chinese-medicine/chinese-medicine

16 www.floridavediccollege.edu/ayurveda/history.htm

17 www.acupuncture.com/education/tcmbasics/whatisherb.htm

18 everygreenherb.com/shortHistory.html

19 wayneadam.hubpages.com/hub/Medieval-Folk-Medicine

20 www.thenaturalguide.com/natural-medicine-suppression.htm

21 www.uab.edu/reynolds/histfigs/flexner

22 www.naturalnews.com/031332_medical_monopoly_history.html

23 www.discoveriesinmedicine.com/Ni-Ra/Penicillin.html

24 www.healingcancernaturally.com/medical-history.html

25 www.naturalnews.com/027104_cancer_WHO_Chi.html

26 Profectcamelot.org/hoxsey.html

[27] www.tldp.com/issue/166/166hoxs.htm

[28] www.chiro.org/Wilk/

[29] www.fda.gov/Drugs/ResourcesForYou/SpecialFeatures/ucm319379.htm

[30] www.pimatisiwin.com/online/wp-content/uploads/2011/08/07Shroff.pdf

[31] Petersen, Melody. *Our Daily Meds.* NY: Sarah Crichton Books, 2009: p137-140.

[32] www.prwatch.org/node/7026

[33] www.naturalnews.com/010315.html

[34] clinicaltrials.gov/ct2/info/understand

[35] Gordon, MD, James S. "Holistic Medicine: Toward A New Medical Model." *J Clin Psychiatry.* 1981; 42(3); p114-119

CHAPTER 2, Interview with Dr. John Rush

1 Rush, PhD, John A. *An Anthropological Perspective of the Occult.* Berkeley, CA: Frog Books, 1974

2 Rush, PhD, John A. *The Way We Communicate.* Shelburne Falls, MA: Humanity Publications, 1976

3 Rush, PhD, John A. *Clinical Anthropology: An Application of Anthropological Concepts within Clinical Settings.* Westport, CT: Praeger Publishers, 1996

4 Rush, PhD, John A. *Stress and Emotional Health: Applications of Clinical Anthropology,* Westport, CT: Auburn House,1999

5 Rush, PhD, John A. *Failed God: Fractured Myth in a Fragile World.* Berkeley, CA: Frog Books, 2008

6 Rush, PhD, John A. *The Mushroom in Christian Art: The Identity of Jesus in the Development of Christianity.* Berkeley, CA: Frog Books, 2011

7 jeffsekerak.wordpress.com/2010/03/22/legit-alternative-cures-suppressed-by-ama/

CHAPTER 3

[36] www.rmbarry.com/research/natural_medicine.html

[37] www.naturalnews.com/001298.html

[38] www.naturalmedicineoc.com/Testimonials.htm

[39] www.columbia.edu/cu/biology/courses/w4200/pillfreveryill.pdf

[40] www.pharmacytimes.com/news/Pharmacists-Are-Among-the-Most-Trusted-Professionals-Says-Survey

[41] www.lifehack.org/articles/lifestyle/mister-doctor-or-does-it-matter.html

[42] www.nakedcapitalism.com/2007/04/are-doctors-overrated.html

[43] www.commondreams.org/view/2011/01/25-6

[44] www.webmd.com/a-to-z-guides/features/alternative-medicine-integrative-medicine

CHAPTER 4

[45] www.articlesfactory.com/articles/health/how-to-keep-your-body-in-balance.html

[46] hyperphysics.phy-astr.gsu.edu/hbase/thermo/heatreg.html

[47] www.kidsgrowth.com/resources/articledetail.cfm?id=30

[48] medical-dictionary.thefreedictionary.com/chronic+inflammation

[49] www.naturalnews.com/037224_conventional_medicine_chronic_illness_treatment.html

[50] www.ama-assn.org/amednews/2007/03/26/hll20326.htm

[51] www.ncbi.nlm.nih.gov/pubmedhealth/PMH0001467/

[52] sideeffectsbase.com/prednisone-side-effects/

[53] www.diabetes.org/diabetes-basics/diabetes-statistics/

[54] www.cdc.gov/diabetes/pubs/pdf/ndfs_2011.pdf

[55] diabetes.webmd.com/

[56] www.drugs.com/pro/metformin.html

[57] www.drugs.com/pro/actos.html

[58] www.drugs.com/glipizide.html

[59] diabetes.webmd.com/guide/diabetes-causes

[60] www.cdc.gov/diabetes/pubs/pdf/ndfs_2011.pdf

[61] history1900s.about.com/od/medicaladvancesissues/a/penicillin.htm

[62] www.biologie.uni-hamburg.de/b-online/library/history/flemin.html

[63] www.nia.nih.gov/health/publication/biology-aging/immune-system-can-your-immune-system-still-defend-you-you-age

[64] dhhs.ne.gov/publichealth/Pages/ars_general_info_antibi.aspx

[65] www.livingshamanically.com/index.php/living-shamanically/livingshamanically2/living-in-harmony-with-nature-3

CHAPTER 5

[66] Anderson, Richard, ND. *Cleanse and Purify Thyself.* Medford, Oregon: Christobe Publishing, 1988

[67] www.usatoday.com/news/nation/2008-03-10-drugs-tap-water_N.htm

[68] www.immunesystemetc.com/Toxins.html

[69] www.chemicalbodyburden.org/whatisbb.htm

[70] themastercleanse.org

[71] altmedicine.about.com/od/popularhealthdiets/a/Raw_Food.htm

[72] www.optimumhealth.org/

[73] altmedicine.about.com/od/detoxcleansing/a/juice_fasting.htm

[74] www.thenaturalguide.com/detoxification.htm

CHAPTER 6

[75] www.who.int/topics/obesity/en/

[76] www.who.int/mediacentre/factsheets/fs311/en/

[77] fatfacts.pbworks.com/w/page/6734330/Dieting%20Statistics

[78] www.medicinenet.com/script/main/art.asp?articlekey=63586

[79] www.who.int/nutrition/topics/obesity/en/

[80] www.pph-news.com/html/fenphen.html

[81] www.nytimes.com/1999/10/08/business/fen-phen-maker-to-pay-billions-in-settlement-of-diet-injury-cases.html?pagewanted=all

[82] www.fda.gov/Drugs/DrugSafety/PostmarketDrugSafetyInformationforPatientsandProviders/ucm180078.htm

[83] fenphen.org/fen-phen-history

[84] ezinearticles.com/?Using-Thyroid-Hormones-for-Weight-Loss&id=424033

[85] www.webmd.com/diet/news/20101008/fda-rejects-weight-loss-drug-meridia

[86] loss-weightnow.com/Alli_Diet_Pilll.html

[87] www.fda.gov/Drugs/DrugSafety/PostmarketDrugSafetyInformationforPatientsandProviders/ucm213038.htm

[88] nccam.nih.gov/health/hoodia

[89] www.naturalnews.com/030968_hCG_diet_dangers.html

[90] thetimes-tribune.com/news/health-science/research-in-europe-shows-lap-band-outcomes-poor-1.1122804

[91] Kelly, Dr. Gregory. *Shape Shift*. Las Vegas, NV: Health Coach Publishing Company, 2010

[92] www.oa.org/newcomers/twelve-steps/

[93] www.Alfonsoderose.com

## CHAPTER 7

[94] www.medicinenet.com/pain_management/page2.htm

[95] DiPiro, JT, Talbert, RL. *Pharmacotherapy, A Pathophysiologic Approach*. Stanford, CT: Appleton & Lange, 1997

[96] www.mayoclinic.com/health/pain-and-depression/AN01449

[97] www.medicinenet.com/nonsteroidal_antiinflammatory_drugs/page2.htm#side%20effects

[98] www.americanacupuncture.com/killer_cortisone.html

[99] www.drugs.com/morphine.html

[100] eft.mercola.com/

[101] www.exploremeditation.com/meditation-explained/

[102] www.acupuncture.com/education/theory/acuintro.htm

[103] www.dahnyoga.com/about_dahn_yoga/

## CHAPTER 8

[104] www.vilistus.com/bio.shtml

[105] latimesblogs.latimes.com/lanow/2010/12/debi-austin-smoking-through-hole-in-throat.html

[106] dictionary.reference.com/browse/placebo

[107] www.skepdic.com/placebo.html

[108] healthland.time.com/2012/01/18/new-research-on-the-antidepressant-versus-placebo-debate/

[109] www.one-mind-one-energy.com/12-universal-laws.html

[110] www.webmd.com/cancer/default.htm

[111] www.arinanikitina.com/what-is-non-verbal-communication.html

[112] www.minnesotamedicine.com/CurrentIssue/ClinicalJisuMarch2010/tabid/3351/Default.aspx

[113] www.naturalnews.com/010315.html

[114] www.bcmj.org/premise/history-bloodletting

[115] www.toptenz.net/top-10-unhealthy-fad-diets.php

[116] www.trepanationguide.com/history.htm

[117] www.drwaynedyer.com/blog

[118] www.tut.com

## CHAPTER 9

[119] dictionary.reference.com/browse/emotions

[120] www.imshealth.com/imshealth/Global/Content/IMS%20Institute/Documents/IHII_UseOfMed_report%20.pdf

[121] Kessler RC, Chiu WT, Demler O, Walters EE. "Prevalence, severity, and comorbidity of twelve-month DSM-IV disorders in the National Comorbidity Survey Replication (NCS-R)." *Archives of General Psychiatry,* 2005 Jun;62(6):617-27

[122] www.imshealth.com/imshealth/Global/Content/IMS%20Institute/Documents/IHII_UseOfMed_report%20.pdf

[123] www.reuters.com/article/2011/02/04/us-many-get-antidepressants-no-psychiatr-idUSTRE7136EW20110204

[124] www.nimh.nih.gov/health/topics/child-and-adolescent-mental-health/antidepressant-medications-for-children-and-adolescents-information-for-parents-and-caregivers.shtml

[125] biopsychiatry.com/bigpharma/davidhealy.html

[126] www.louisehay.com/

[127] eft.mercola.com/

[128] somaticexperiencing.com/news-and-updates/a-primer-of-somatic-experiencing.html

[129] 12step.org/steps/the-12-steps.html

## CHAPTER 10

[130] www.cancer.org/acs/groups/content/@epidemiologysurveilance/documents/document/acspc-029771.pdf

[131] www.citizenshealth.org/about-legislation.html

[132] medical-dictionary.thefreedictionary.com/chemotherapy

[133] www.cancer.gov/cancertopics/coping/radiation-therapy-and-you/page2

134 altered-states.net/barry/rife/suppression.htm
135 www.naturalnews.com/027104_cancer_WHO_Chi.html
136 www.cancure.org/hoxsey_clinic.htm
137 www.citizenshealth.org/mission.html
138 www.naturalnews.com/027104_cancer_WHO_Chi.html
139 www.msnbc.msn.com/id/30763438/ns/health-childrens_health/t/judge-rules-family-cant-refuse-chemo-boy/
140 miracleii-4u.com/cancer-practitioners-laws.htm
141 www.webmd.com/cancer
142 Campbell, T. Colin & Campbell. *The China Study*. Dallas. Tx: BenBella Books, 2007
143 www.LouiseHay.com
144 www.rife.org/
145 alternativecancer.us/ozone.htm
146 www.cancertutor.com/
147 www.medicalnewstoday.com/releases/12154.php
148 www.1cure4cancer.com/controlcancer/information/laetrile.htm
149 www.naturalnews.com/027020_cancer_AMA_treatment.html#ixzz1bY44ZhZU
150 www.abraham-hicks.com/lawofattractionsource/journal.php?moneyquotes

## CHAPTER 11

151 www.pacode.com/secure/data/049/chapter27/chap27toc.html
152 www.chron.com/news/houston-texas/article/New-rules-ban-gifts-that-drug-companies-can-give-1741785.php
153 money.cnn.com/2011/06/01/news/economy/prescription_drug_abuse/index.htm

## CHAPTER 12

154 www.actos.com/
155 www.nlm.nih.gov/medlineplus/druginfo/meds/a699055.html
156 www.novolog.com/
157 www.lantus.com/
158 www.lantus.com/solostar-insulin-pen/solostar-insulin-pen.aspx
159 www.byetta.com
160 allergies.emedtv.com/claritin/difference-between-clarinex-and-claritin.html
161 www.nlm.nih.gov/medlineplus/druginfo/meds/a601086.html
162 www.aciphex.com/
163 www.drugs.com/clonazepam.html
164 www.drugs.com/celebrex.html
165 www.drugs.com/vicodin.html
166 www.healthline.com/goldcontent/docusate

167 www.vytorin.com/
168 www.drugs.com/temazepam.html
169 www.medicinenet.com/promethazine_and_codeine/article.htm
170 www.procrit.com/
171 www.abilify.com/
172 www.geodon.com/
173 www.drugs.com/flonase.html
174 www.spiriva.com/
175 Trapp & Barnard (2010). "Usefulness of Vegetarian and Vegan Diets for TreatingType 2 Diabetes." *Curr Diab Rep;* 2010, 10:152-158, www.springerlink.com/content/h710625r766h1114/
176 www.nhs.uk/conditions/chronic-obstructive-pulmonary-disease
177 www.chinese-holistic-health-exercises.com/anxiety-breathing-techniques.html
178 www.mayoclinic.com/health/meditation/HQ01070

CHAPTER 13
179 www.ncbi.nlm.nih.gov/pmc/articles/PMC2811591/
180 www.drugs.com/stats/top100/2011/sales
181 www.diabeteshealth.com/read/2010/10/09/6898/the-cost-of-diabetes/
182 www.naturalnews.com/003204.html
183 www.nejm.org/doi/pdf/10.1056/NEJMsa070502
184 www.nejm.org/doi/full/10.1056/NEJMsa070502#t=articleBackground
185 Petersen, Melody. *Our Daily Meds.* New York, NY: Sarah Crichton Books, 2008; pg 50-51
186 Petersen, Melody. *Our Daily Meds.* New York, NY: Sarah Crichton Books, 2008; pg 280
187 Petersen, Melody. *Our Daily Meds.* New York, NY: Sarah Crichton Books, 2008; pg 281
188 www.nap.edu/openbook.php?isbn=0309068371
189 Kohn LT, Corrigan JM, Donaldson MS, eds. *Committee on Quality of Health Care in America, Institute of Medicine. To Err is Human: Building a Safer Health System.* Washington, DC: National Academy Press, 1999
190 Aspden P, Wolcott JA, Bootman JL, Cronenwett LR, eds. *Preventing Medication Errors.* Washington, DC: National Academy Press, 2006
191 US Pharmacopeia. *Summary of Information Submitted to MEDMARX in the year 2002: The Quest for Quality.* Accessed July 2008 www.usp.org.
192 Budnitz DS, Pollock DA, Weidenbach KN, Mendelsohn AB, Schroeder TJ, Annest JL. "National surveillance of emergency department visits for outpatient adverse drug events." *Journal of Medical Association (JAMA),* 2006;296(15):1858-1866,2006
193 Starfield, Barbara. "Is US Health Really the Best in the World?" *Journal of Medical Association (JAMA),* July 2000;284, No4, July 26
194 secure.pharmacytimes.com/lessons/200809-01.asp
195 www.anh-europe.org/news/polypharmacy-increases-risk-of-death-in-over-65s

196 www.fda.gov/Drugs/DrugSafety/
PostmarketDrugSafetyInformationforPatientsandProviders/ucm180078.
htm
197 Petersen, Melody. *Our Daily Meds.* New York, NY: Sarah Crichton Books,
2008; pg 166-72
198 www.pbs.org/newshour/rundown/2010/11/drugmakers-pull-painkillers-
darvon-darvocet-from-market.html
199 en.wikipedia.org/wiki/Quinolone
200 Petersen, Melody. Our Daily Meds. New York, NY: Sarah Crichton Books,
2008; pg 212-17, 243-49
201 www.cbsnews.com/8301-204_162-617223.html
202 dida.library.ucsf.edu/pdf/oha00a10
203 Petersen, Melody. *Our Daily Meds.* New York, NY: Sarah Crichton Books,
2008; pg 49
204 Petersen, Melody. *Our Daily Meds.* New York, NY: Sarah Crichton Books,
2008; pg 179
205 Petersen, Melody. *Our Daily Meds.* New York, NY: Sarah Crichton Books,
2008; pg 180
206 Petersen, Melody. *Our Daily Meds.* New York, NY: Sarah Crichton Books,
2008; pg 327
207 www.fda.gov/ICECI/Inspections/IOM/ucm124442.htm
208 www.drugwatch.com/2012/01/18/fda-black-box-warnings/
209 www.ama-assn.org/amednews/2008/07/28/hlsc0728.htm
210 www.sciencedaily.com/releases/2004/12/041203100252.htm
211 www.ncbi.nlm.nih.gov/books/NBK53952/
212 www.ouralexander.org/war1.htm
213 Petersen, Melody. *Our Daily Meds.* New York, NY: Sarah Crichton Books,
2008; pg 248-9
214 www.ft.com/cms/s/0/af7767ec-4406-11d9-af06-00000e2511c8.
html#axzz2EABVULy

## CHAPTER 14

215 www.naturalnews.com/036702_doctors_nutrition_fatalities.html
216 Adams KE et al. "Status of nutrition education in medical schools."
*American Journal of Clinical Nutrition,* 2006, 83, 4, 941S-944S.
217 Campbell, T. Colin. & Campbell. *The China Study.* Dallas, Tx: BenBella
Books, 2007
218 Swinburn BA, et al. The global obesity pandemic: shaped by global drivers
and local environments. *Lancet.* 2011, 378 (9793), 804-14.
219 Olshansky SJ, et al. "A potential decline in life expectancy in the United
States in the 21st century." *N Engl J Med.* 2005, 352(11), 1138-45.
220 www.citizenshealth.org/
221 lingli.ccer.edu.cn/ahe2011/papers/8/Donohue,%20J.%20M.,%20M.%20
Cevasco,%20et%20al.%20%282007%29.pdf
222 www.anh-europe.org/campaigns/freedom-health-choice.
223 www.anh-europe.org/
224 www.anh-europe.org/documents/risk-relative-to-legal-dietary-supplements

CHAPTER 15

[225] mariaerving.com/how-to-use-the-abraham-hicks-emotional-guidance-scale/

[226] www.abraham-hicks.com/lawofattractionsource/index.php

[227] www.healyourlife.com/author-louise-l-hay/2010/01/wisdom/personal-growth/do-you-give-your-power-away

[228] www.ariseandshine.com/books/cleanse-purify-thyself-book-1.html

[229] Phillips, Brent. *Where Science Meets Spirit: The Formula for Miracles.* Los Angeles, CA 2008

[230] mayibefrankmovie.com/